SEXY LEGS

HOW TO GET THEM & HOW TO KEEP THEM

James A. Peterson, Ph.D.
Susan L. Peterson

LEISURE PRESS

NEW YORK

A publication of
Leisure Press
597 Fifth Avenue; New York, N.Y. 10017

Library of Congress Catalog Card Number: 83-90741

ISBN: 0-88011-162-3

Cover and book design: Brian Groppe
Production: John Jett
Cover photographs: David Madison
All text photographs by
Tim Davis, except as noted:
Wayne Glusker: 3
Janeart: 7
David Madison: 8
Movie Star News: 5
Gene Rockey: 4
Typesetting: Lewis Publishing; Oakland, California

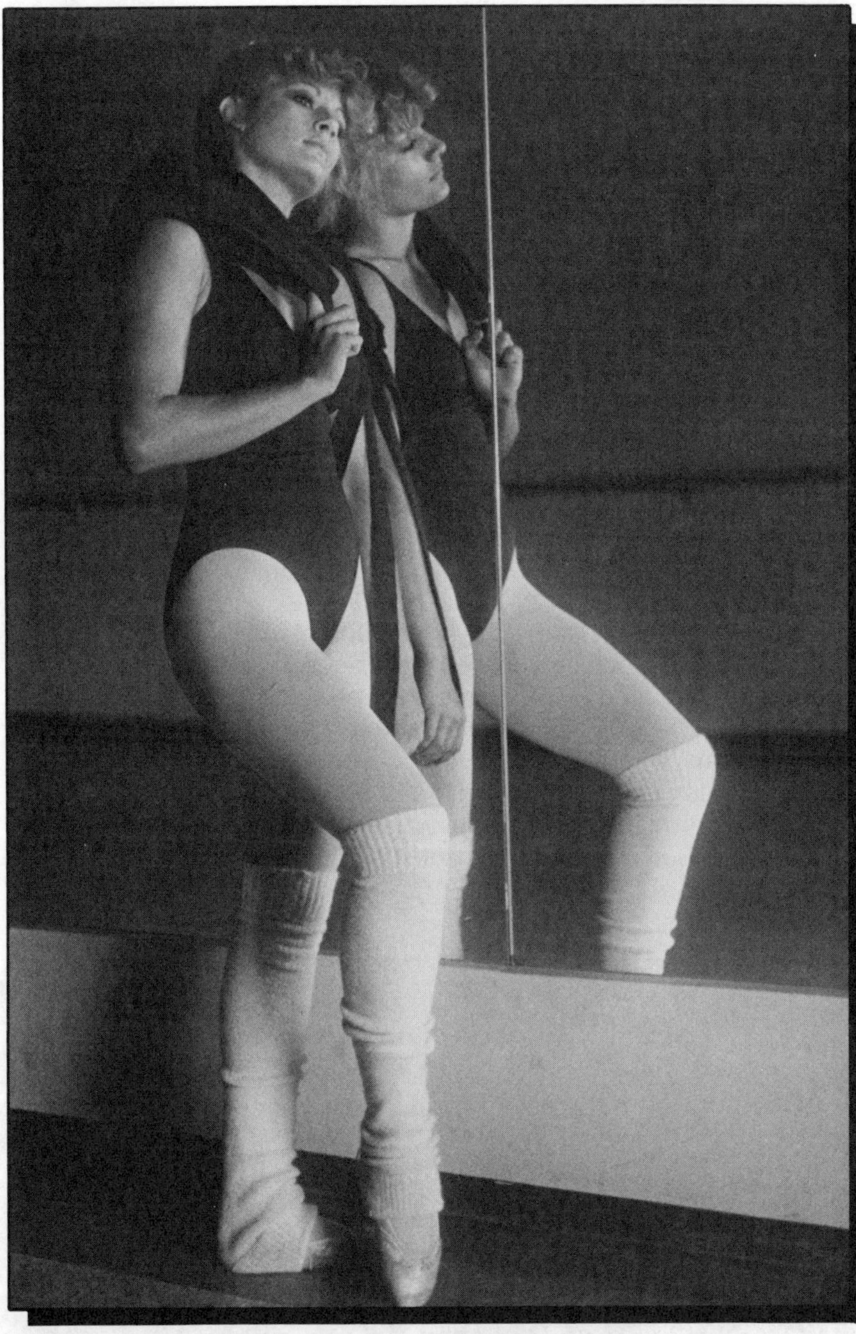

Your sexy legs are just weeks away!

Legs. They support us. They propel us. They carry us. They lift us. In other words, they play a critical role in our lives. We ask a lot of them and they seldom let us down. Somewhat paradoxically, we expect our legs to look "great" in addition to all the work they perform. Some people, however, don't like the "look" of their legs. Not surprisingly, legs come in all sizes and shapes: fat ones, thin ones, stocky ones, shapely ones, firm ones, and so on. Since you purchased this book on firming up and shaping your legs, obviously you've decided that yours are somewhat less than as sexy as you'd like them to be.

Before you read too much further, however, we feel it is only fair to warn you that you're facing a good news/bad news situation. The good news is that almost anyone can develop sexy legs. The bad news is that it requires work . . . and patience. There is no magic pill that will enable you to acquire sexy legs overnight, no supernatural spell that will give you the will power to do what is necessary to whip your legs into shape. All anyone can do for you is to give you the information on how to develop sexy legs. What you do with that information is up to you.

The exercises in this book—when combined with sensible eating habits—will develop your legs to a degree perhaps beyond your wildest imagination. The shapely, firm, sexy legs you've always wanted are yours for the asking if you're willing to work for them. No one else can perform the exercises for you. You must do them . . .correctly, regularly and diligently. If you compromise the proper way of doing the exercises, you'll compromise your goal of having sexy legs.

Remember, sexy is in. Think sexy. Your sexy legs are just weeks away.

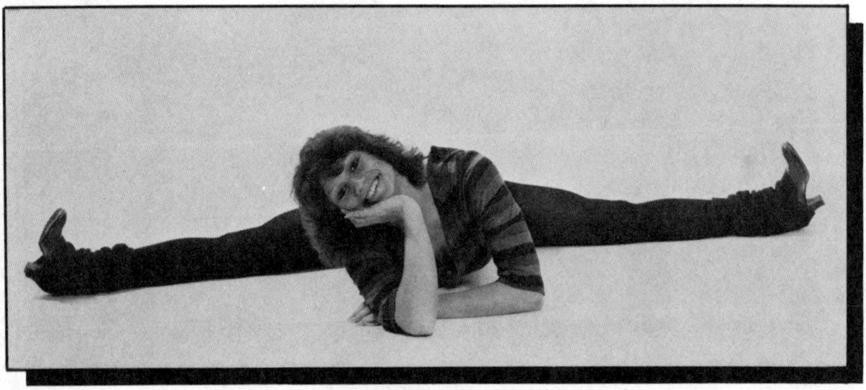

Sexy is in. Think sexy. Firm, shapely legs are sexy!

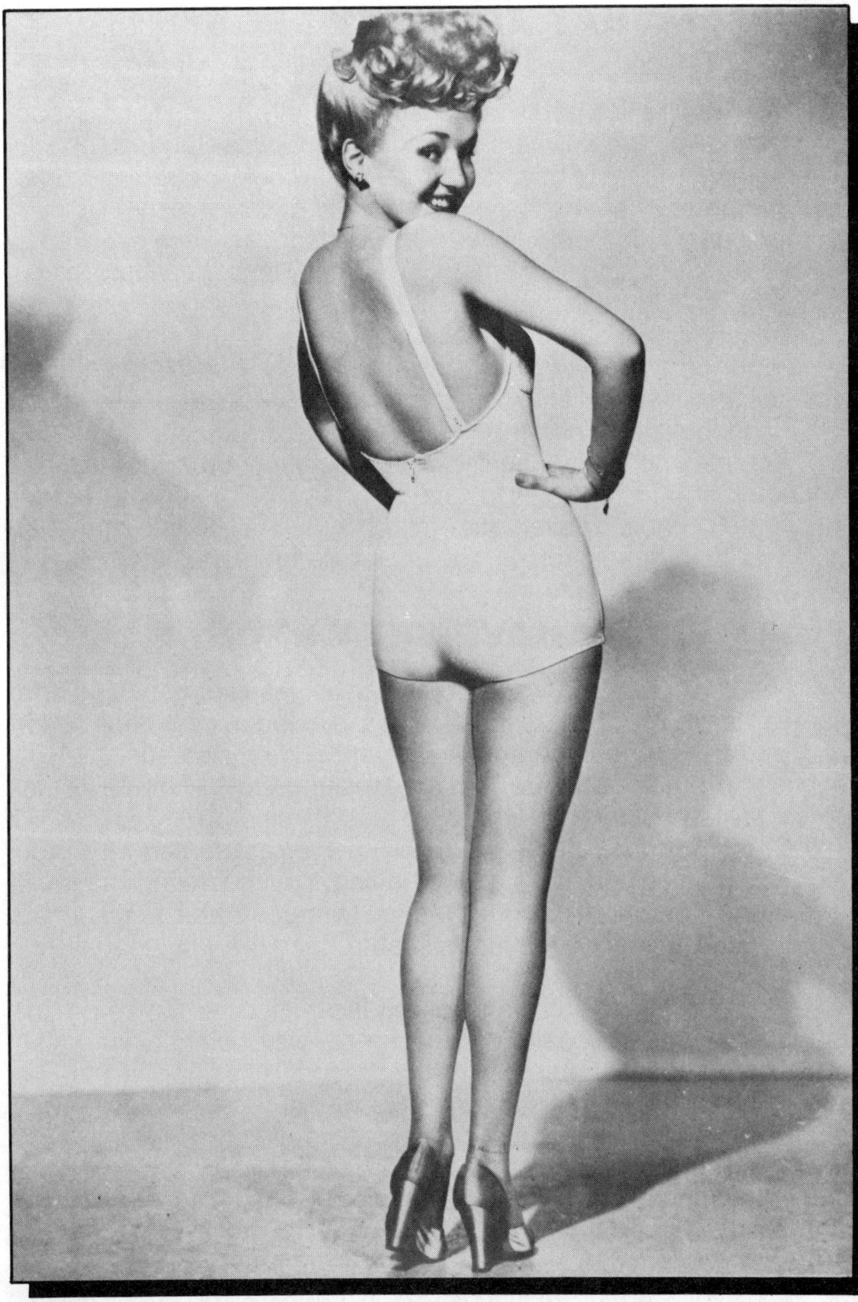

Sexy legs can have a positive effect on both your physical health and mental well-being.

WHAT ARE SEXY LEGS?

Sexy legs have several characteristics. They're firm and shapely. They usually belong to *other* people. They allow their owners (of sexy legs) to wear the clothes they want without regard to how well those clothes hide protruding bulges. They're the envy of all the owner's friends. If you have them, they're usually worth a kind word or two from your spouse when exposed by shorts or a swimming suit. But above all, sexy legs contribute to your sense of physical and mental well-being.

Beauty, as the old adage goes, is in the eye of the beholder. If you think your legs are sexy, then they're sexy. If you feel good about yourself, that's super. That's also what this book is all about—feeling good and looking terrific.

You may be wondering if it is necessary for you to look like Loni Anderson or Burt Reynolds to have sexy legs. Emphatically no! Sexy legs are attainable by everyone—short people, tall people, brunettes, blondes, red heads, older adults, teenagers, you, us . . . literally everyone.

WHY HAVE SEXY LEGS?

Unfortunately, some people don't have a "leg to stand on" when it comes to being healthy, looking terrific, and feeling good about themselves. The reason—unsightly fat deposits on their legs. Are these deposits good for you? No! Can these fat transplants be firmed up and eliminated? Yes! . . . but it takes work on your part. Is it worth the effort? Yes! Surplus fat on your legs is a drain on your physical well-being. Your heart and other bodily systems are forced to work overtime to support what is essentially dead weight. Eliminate the fat and you reduce the work load of your heart, your lungs, etc.

The other reason for wanting sexy legs—and certainly as important as your physical health—is your mental well-being. It is important to feel good about yourself. Let's face it, ours is basically a thin-is-in oriented society. Both visual and print media — television, movies, magazines, newspapers, etc.—hammer that point incessantly. Thin is *the* look. Thin people are portrayed as glamorous, sociable, well-liked, intelligent, contemporary, opportunistic . . . in a word, successful.

No one wants to feel unsuccessful. And no one wants to feel self-conscious about their looks. Who needs anxieties over what clothing is appropriate for public places? Who wants to worry about which public places (e.g. the beach, tennis court, etc.) are least likely to be embarassing?. Build your self-confidence—give yourself a "leg to stand on." Develop those sexy legs—NOW!

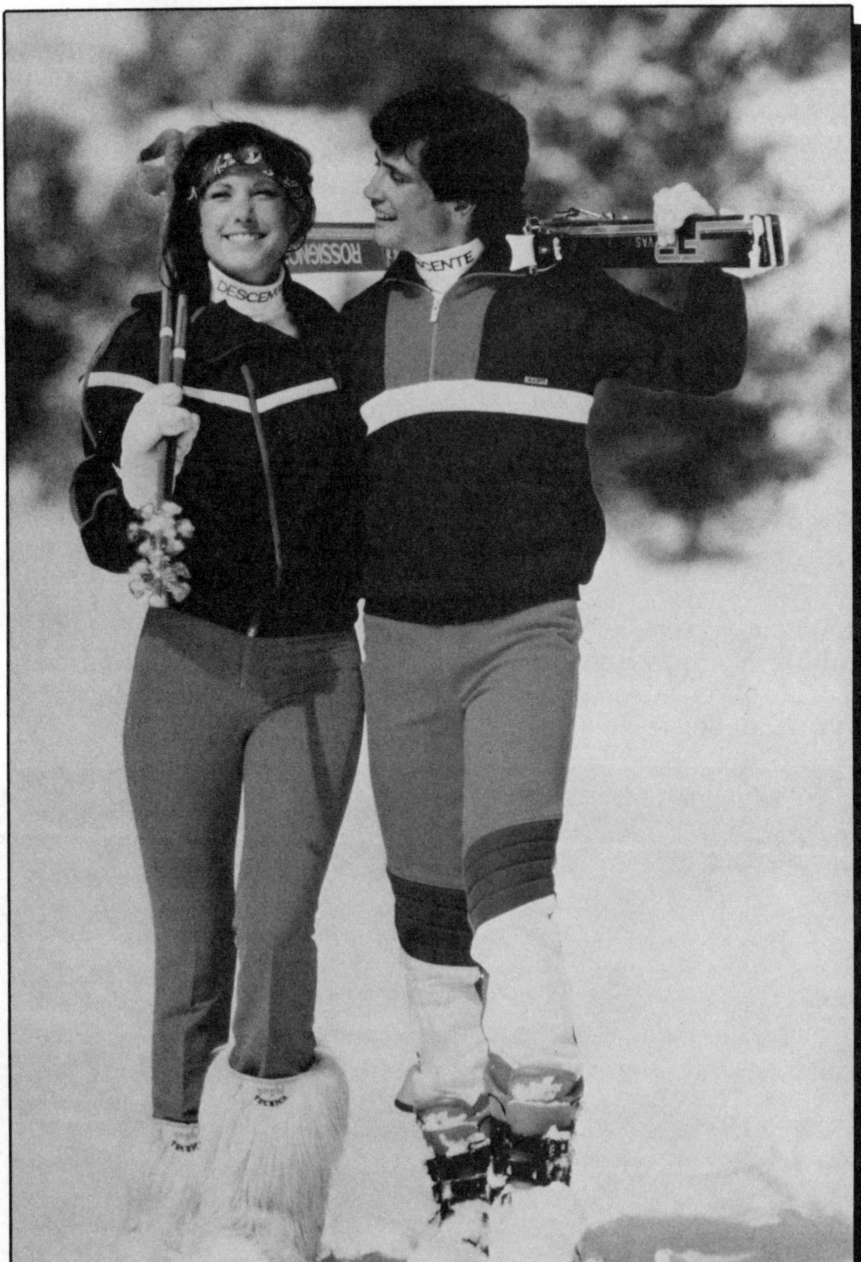

Sexy legs can help everyone feel good and look terrific.

THE PROGRAM

OK! OK! So we convinced you. Now what? You've already taken the critical first step—you've recognized the need to shape up your legs. You've also taken the logical second step by obtaining accurate advice (the steps, exercises and programs described in this book) on how to accomplish your goal of overhauling your leg muscles.

The next step is to identify what exercises to do and "put on your exercising shoes to beat the flabby legs blues." Before you get started, however, (the exercises are described and illustrated in the next section of this book) we'd like to provide you with a few basic guidelines to follow in order to insure that your program will give you the greatest possible results, in the least amount of required time and in the safest possible manner.

EXERCISE GUIDELINES

1 Before beginning any exercise program, you should have a medical examination by a physician. Be sure to inform your physician of your intention to exercise. If an injury occurs or you become ill during your exercise program, consult your physician before continuing.

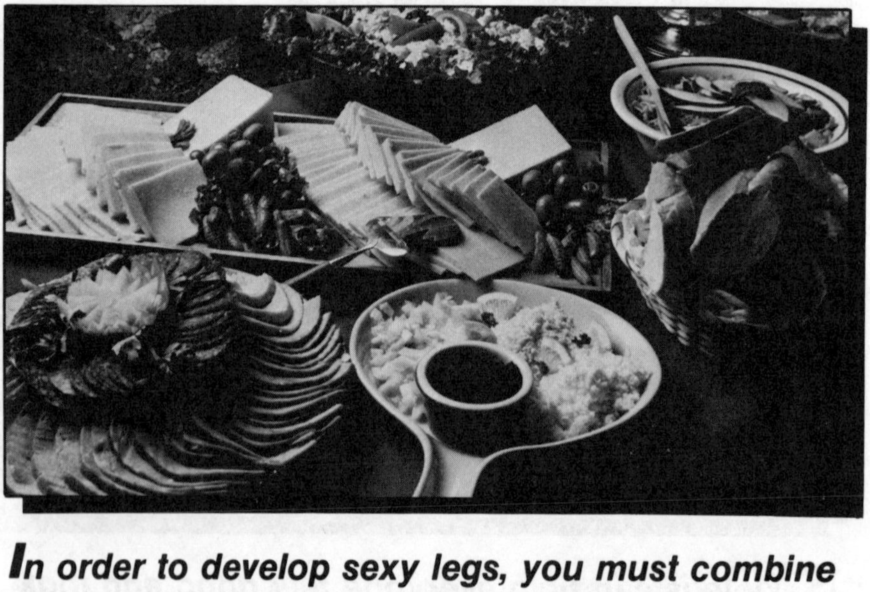

In order to develop sexy legs, you must combine your exercise program with sensible eating habits.

2 The time of day to exercise is an individual matter. However, it would be wise to wait at least an hour after eating before exercising.

3 What you wear, where you exercise, and whether you exercise with another person or alone are all personal decisions. It is in your best interest to make these decisions prior to starting your exercise program if possible.

4 Try to exercise at least 4 to 5 times a week. If you exercise regularly, you should see substantial improvement within a month. Remember, the more you exercise, the quicker the improvement will be. Be patient, however. You didn't get out of shape overnight and you won't get into shape overnight.

5 You will achieve better results from these exercises if you perform them slowly and smoothly. Fast, jerky movement are ballistic. Such movements are counterproductive to your goal of achieving sexy legs. When you exercise ballistically, your muscles are not required to work throughout their full range of motion for each exercise. Literally, in this instance, you're merely throwing your body, not exercising it. When you perform exercises in a fast, jerky manner, you're also increasing your chances of being injured.

6 Be careful not to arch your back (hyperextend) while performing those exercises which involve your lower back. If at all possible, always try to keep your lower back straight or stable while exercising. The majority of the sexy leg exercises are done from a seated or floor position rather than from a standing position. This is because exercises performed from a seated or prone position generally place less strain on your lower back. Since millions of people suffer from back problems, it is important for the back to be protected as much as possible while exercising. In addition, the *best* leg exercises are performed from a seated or prone position rather than from a standing position!

7 While reading the directions for performing each exercise, be sure to pay special attention to the "notes" written for certain exercises. All directions should be followed closely so that you perform every exercise correctly. Remember, if you compromise the way an exercise should be done, you compromise the results that you can achieve.

8 Your exercise program should include both warm-up and warm-down exercises, in addition to the leg exercises.

9 Under normal circumstances, your exercise routine should take at least 15 to 20 minutes including warm-ups and warm-downs. Remember, don't be in a hurry while exercising your leg muscles. You must perform the exercise properly if your program is to be both effective and safe.

10 Although exercising should not be painful, you may experience sore leg muscles the first few days of your program. Do not quit exercising. Continue, but at a slower pace; use fewer repetitions, at a different level, etc. Under no circumstances, however, should you eliminate your warm-ups and warm-downs from your workout. They're important. Do them every workout. A warm bath or shower may also be helpful. Keep in mind that although it may seem like a lifetime, muscle soreness will only last for a few days. If for some reason it lasts longer, either your program is much too strenuous or you may have a medical problem which requires attention. Usually, it's your program. In that instance, you'll have to adjust it accordingly.

11 The quickest way to attain sexy legs is to combine exercise with sensible eating habits. Exercise alone may not be enough. In fact, to lose pounds you generally need to both diet and exercise.

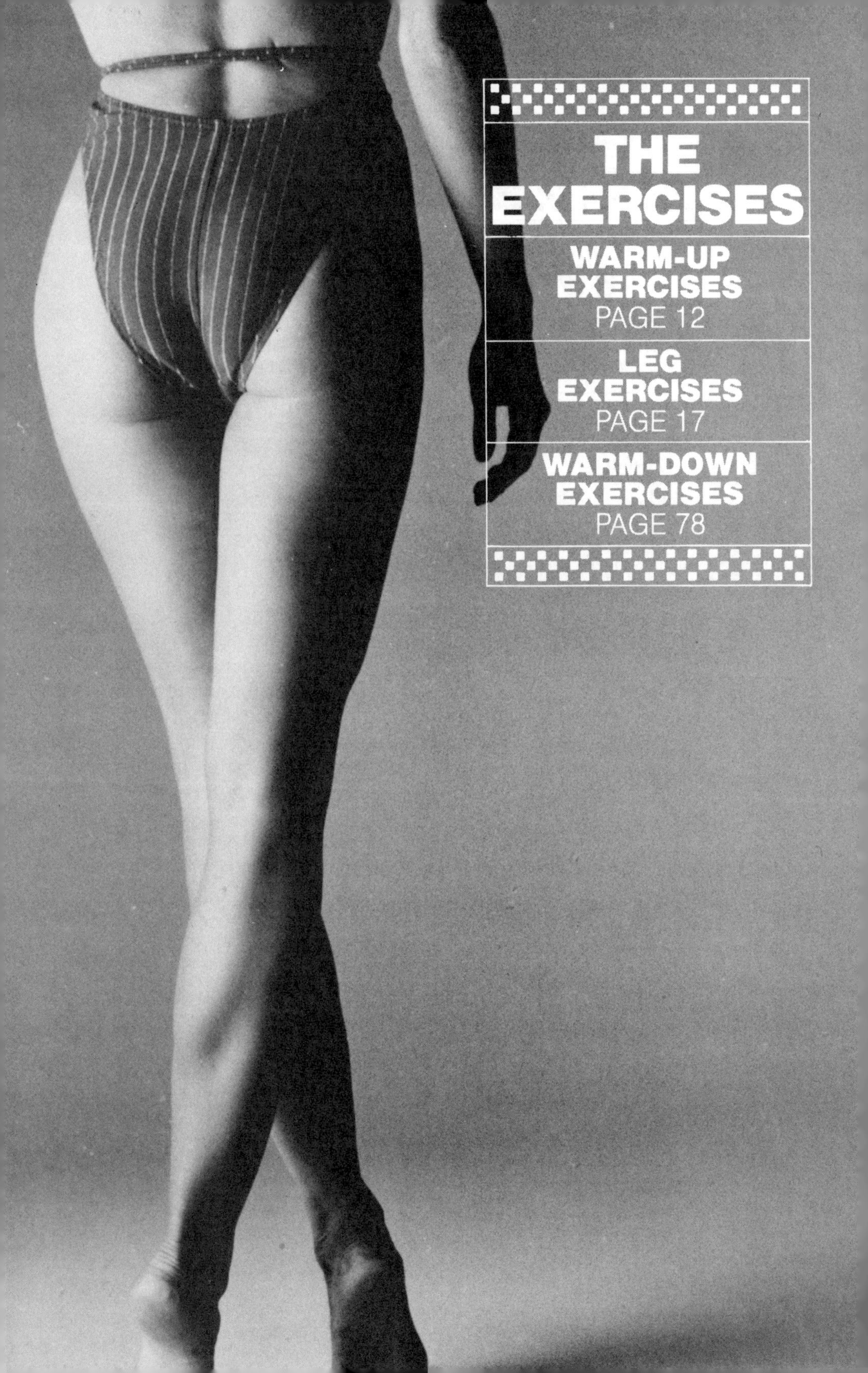

THE EXERCISES

WARM-UP EXERCISES*

Warm-up exercises are intended to increase your circulation and raise the temperature in your muscles. They should be performed at the beginning of every exercise workout to prepare your body for strenuous activity. The primary objective of warm-ups is to prevent injury. Since the leg muscles are particularly susceptible to strains and pulls (often caused by a lack of proper warm-up and stretching), it is very important that you perform these warm-ups prior to doing the various leg exercises found throughout this book. They are designed to stretch all the major muscle groups found in the legs.

All of the suggested warm-up exercises should be performed slowly and smoothly. Do not bounce or jerk while stretching. The amount of time you should spend on warm-ups is up to you. We recommend, however, that you devote at least 5 minutes to the warm-up portion of your routine. While stretching, you should place a mild stretch on the muscle and *hold* that stretch without forcing the muscle to be overstretched. Most stretches should be held for 6 to 10 seconds or longer (from 30 to 60 seconds) if you choose to do only a couple of repetitions. Generally, 4 to 6 repetitions will be sufficient. The exact number of repetitions and specific exercises you do, however, is an individual choice.

---

*Additional information as well as stretching exercises may be found in *The Woman's Stretching Book* by Susan L. Peterson, Leisure Press, 1983. The following warm-up exercises are taken from that book.

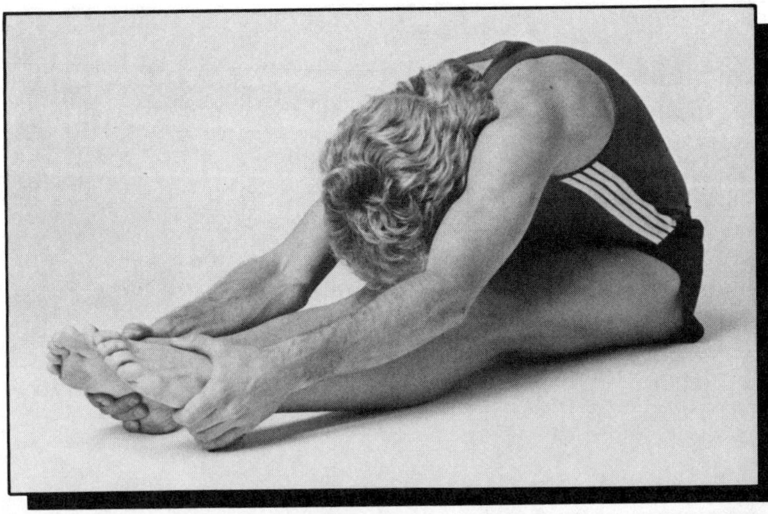

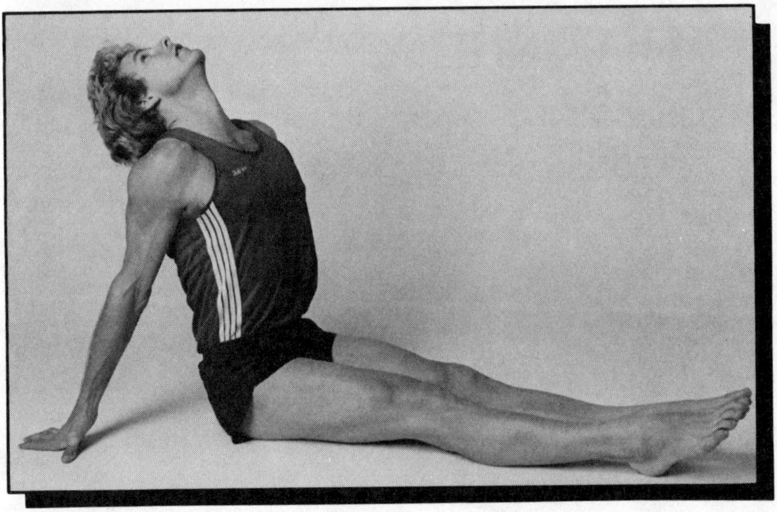

1

Seated—Legs Together: (Position 1) Sit with both legs together and extended with your feet relaxed. Slowly lean forward from the hips and reach both your hands toward your feet. Hold the stretch, then return to the sitting position. Continue stretching (Position 2) by placing your hands on the floor behind you, and look up to the ceiling while arching your back *very slightly*. Hold this stretch, then return to the sitting position, Position 1, etc. *Note:* If you are unable to reach your ankles or your feet, just reach and stretch as far as possible.

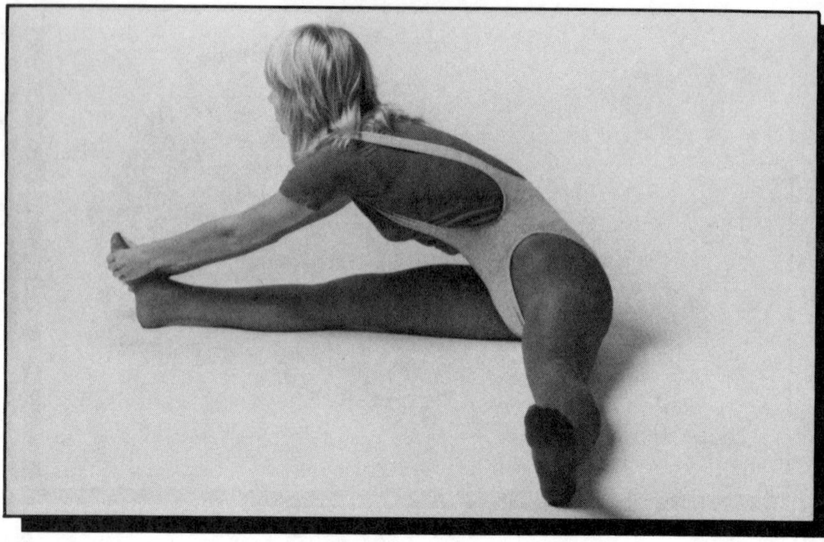

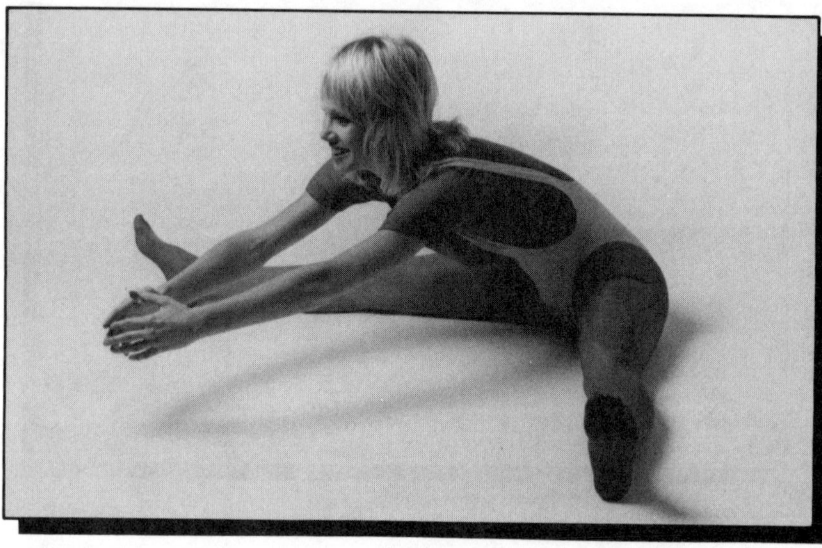

2

Seated—Legs Apart: Sit with both legs apart and your feet relaxed (Position 1). Turn to your right, lean forward from your hips, and reach with both hands toward your right foot. Hold the stretch, return to the straight sitting position (Position 2). Then repeat the stretch by reaching both hands forward toward the floor. Hold this stretch, and finally, (Position 3) reach both hands to your left foot. Hold, then repeat the sequence right, center, left, etc.

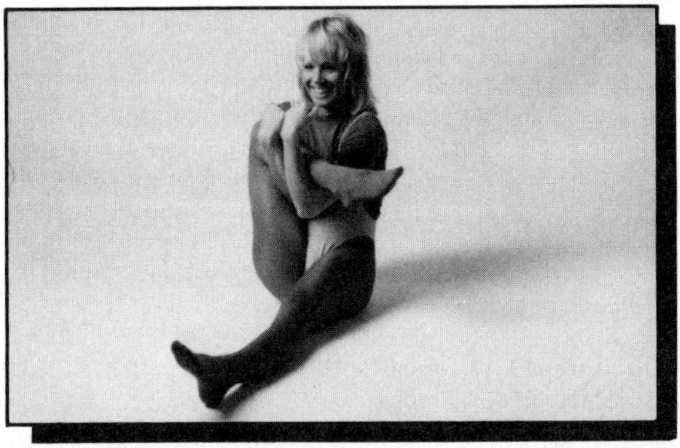

3

Seated Hip Stretch: Sit with your left leg extended along the floor, bend your right leg across your body to the left and pull your calf toward you with both arms wrapped around your lower leg. You may want to lean slightly backward for an additional stretch. Hold, relax and repeat with your other leg. Continue to switch right, left, etc.

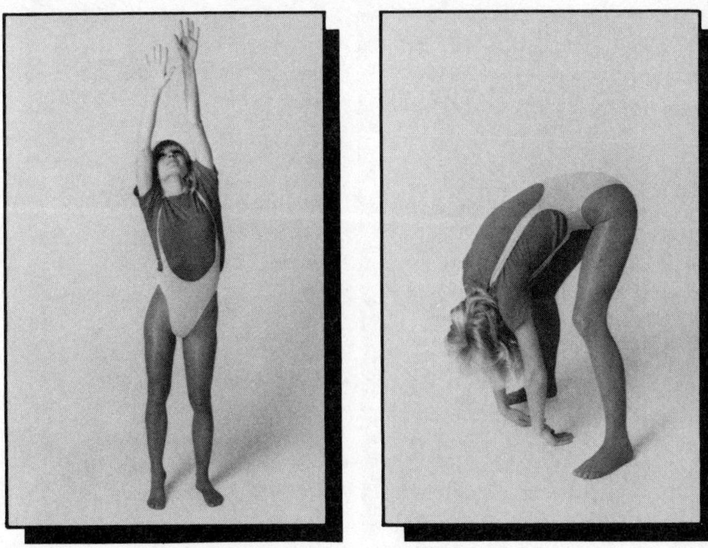

4

Standing Reach Up and Down: Stand with your legs apart. Look up to the ceiling and reach both hands upward for several counts (stand on your toes for an added stretch). Slowly bend forward and relax for several counts. Bend your knees slightly so that the stretch is not so intense. Slowly curl upward to return to the standing position and repeat the reach.

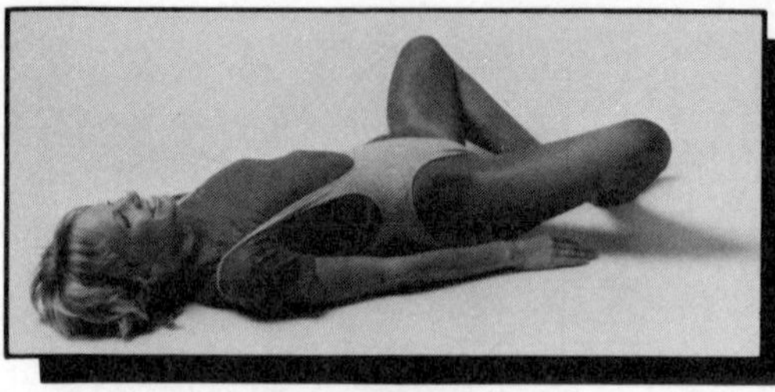

5

Groin Stretch: Lie on your back with your arms extended at your sides. Bend both your knees and put the bottom of your feet together—letting your knees fall to the outside towards the floor. Hold that position, relax and repeat.

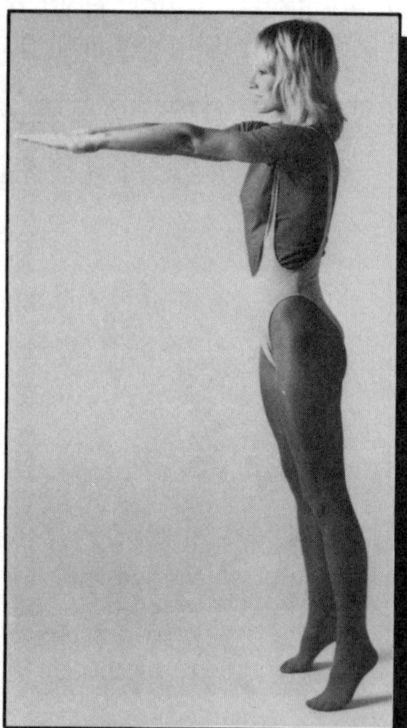

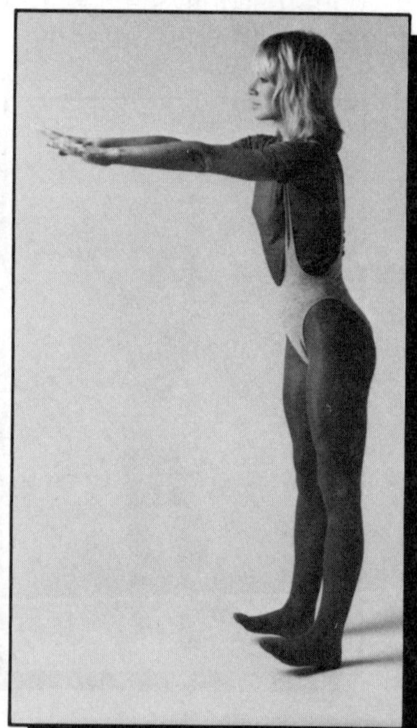

6

Standing Toe Balance: Stand with your legs slightly apart and your arms held straight out in front of you for balance *or* you may place both hands on a wall or chair back for balance. Now raise up onto your toes, then rock back onto your heels. Repeat in succession toes, heels, etc.

LEG EXERCISES

These exercises are divided into three groups. Level #I exercises are designed for those individuals who are unaccustomed to strenuous exercise involving the leg muscles. Level II exercises are slightly more difficult than Level I exercises and should be performed by those individuals with an intermediate level of leg muscle fitness. The most strenuous level of exercises is Level III—the level for advanced performers.

Your basic exercise program should include a minimum of at least 8 exercises at each intensity level (I, II, or III). We recommend that when you are initially performing the exercises at a particular intensity level, you do 6 to 8 repetitions of each exercise. Once you successfully complete 10 to 12 repetitions of most exercises at Level I, you can move up to Level II, or from Level II to Level III if you can comfortably do 10 to 12 repetitions of most of the Level II exercises.

LEVEL I: THE BEGINNER

1

SIDE LYING KNEE BEND

Lie on your side with one leg on top of the other. Support your upper body with one hand held under your head and the other placed on the floor in front of you. Lift your right leg 4 to 6" upward and quickly bend your right knee up toward your chest, pause and then extend your leg to the starting position. Repeat the knee bend in succession. Repeat the exercise on your other side with your left knee.

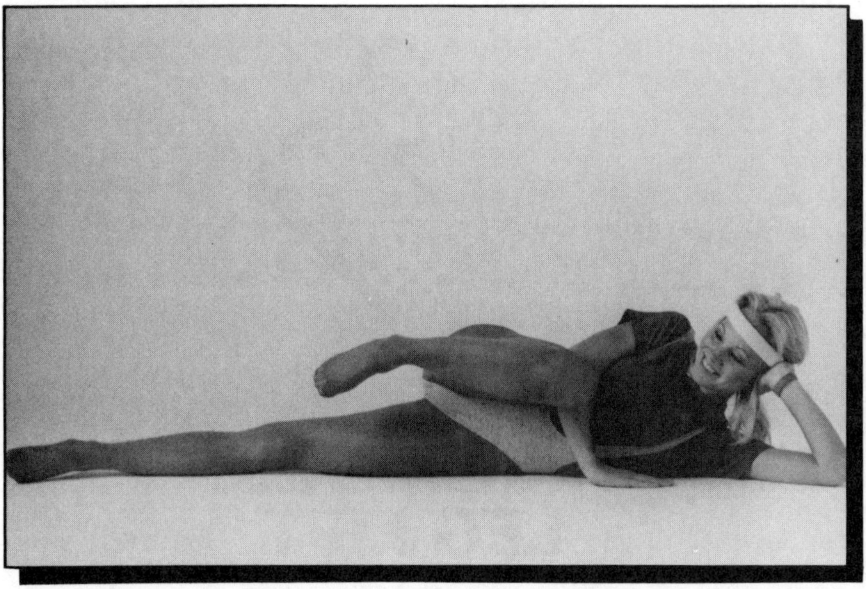

2

HAND-KNEE LEG LIFT

Kneel on your hands and knees. Extend your right leg backward along the floor with your toes pointed. Lift your right leg upward slowly about 12 to 15″ (approximately hip level), pause and slowly lower your leg to touch the floor. Continue lifting and lowering in succession. Repeat the exercise with your left leg. *Note:* Keep your back straight and your head up throughout the exercise.

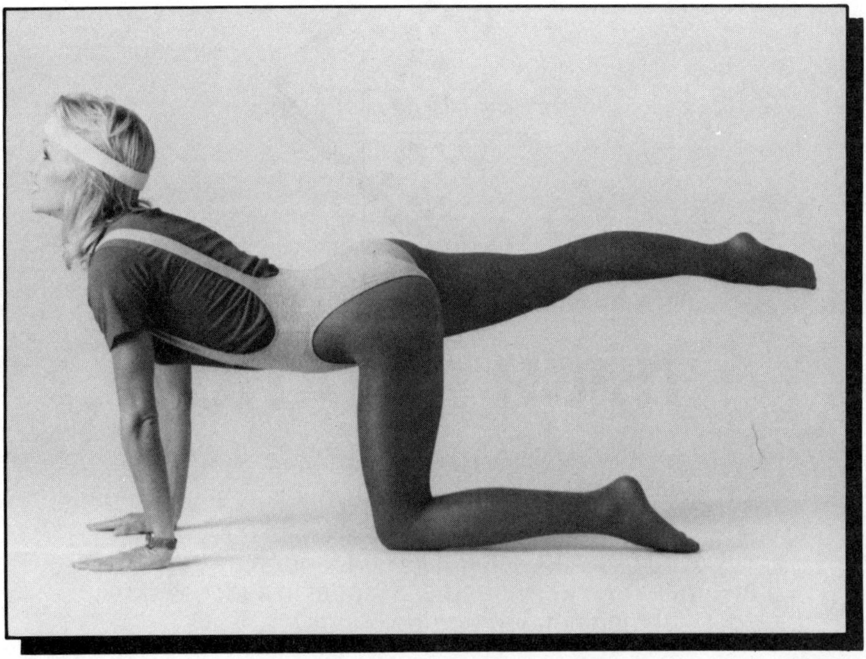

3

THIGH ROTATION

Lie on your back with your arms resting down at your sides, your legs slightly apart and your toes pointed. Slowly rotate your right leg inward and then outward. Repeat this rotation with your left leg, and then both legs together. Repeat in succession with your right leg, left leg and both legs.

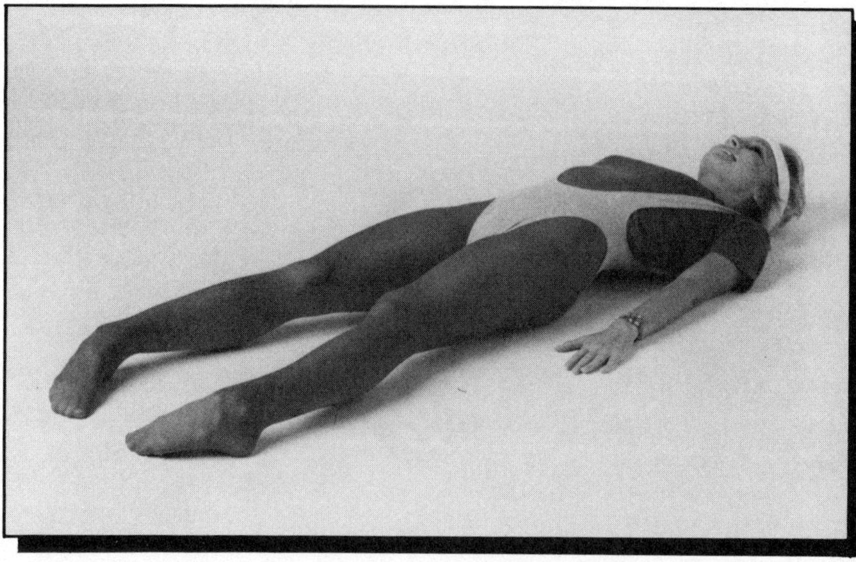

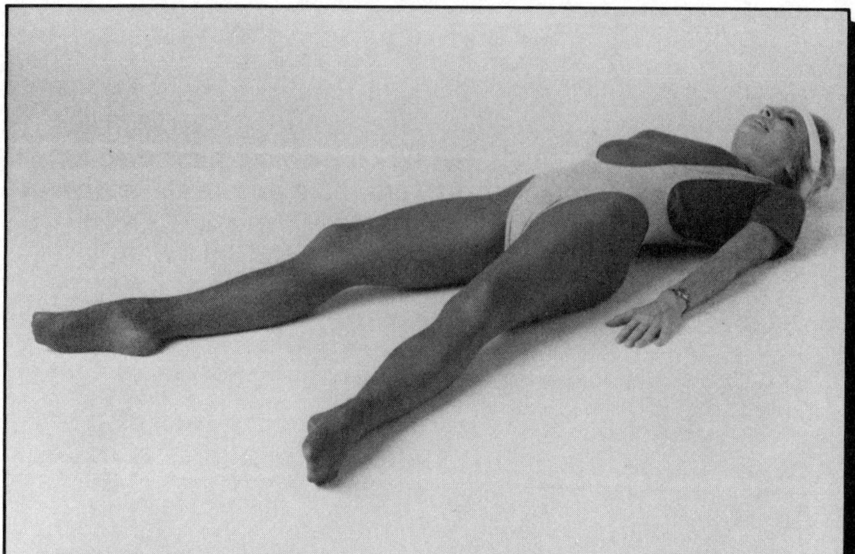

4

SEATED FOOT POINT

Sit with your legs slightly apart and your hands resting on the floor behind you. Slowly point your feet forward, hold and relax. Then slowly point your feet back up toward your shins, hold and relax. Repeat pointing forward and backward in succession.

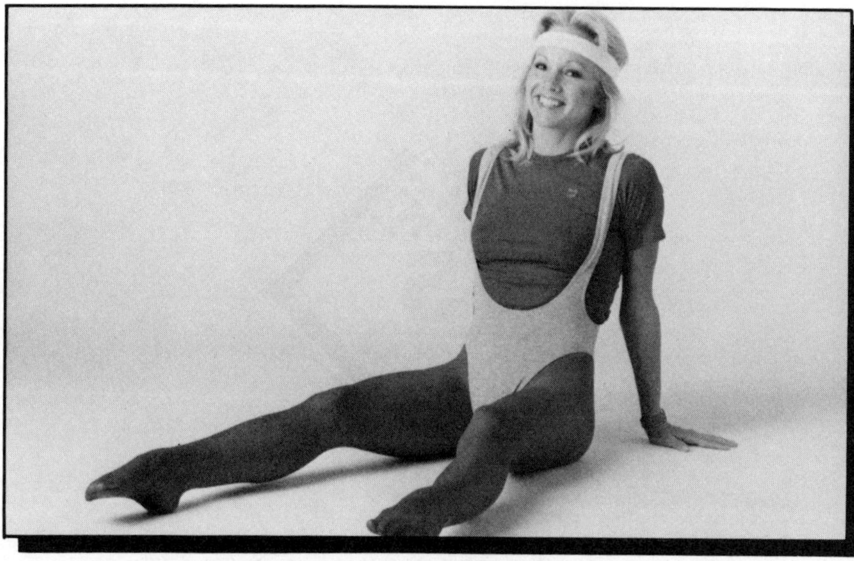

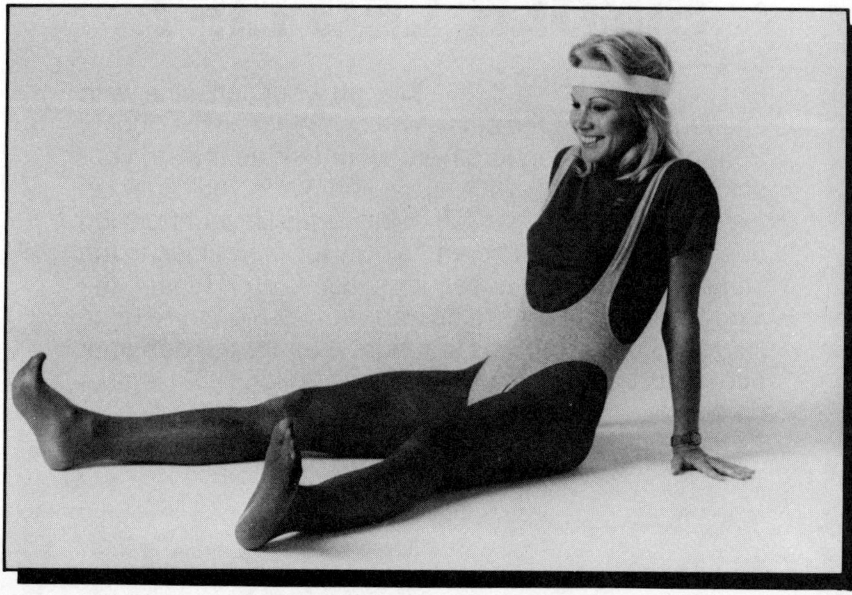

5

SIDE LYING SINGLE LEG LIFT

Lie on your left side with one leg on top of the other, and one hand on the floor in front of you for support. Bend your feet up toward your shins (do not point your toes), and place your right big toe slightly behind your left heel. Slowly lift your right leg upward 8 to 10″, pause and slowly lower your leg to the starting position. Repeat in succession. Repeat the exercise on your other side with your left leg. *Note:* Try to lift very slowly and not too high. Also try to keep your body in a straight line on the floor while lifting your legs — do not let your hips roll forward or backward.

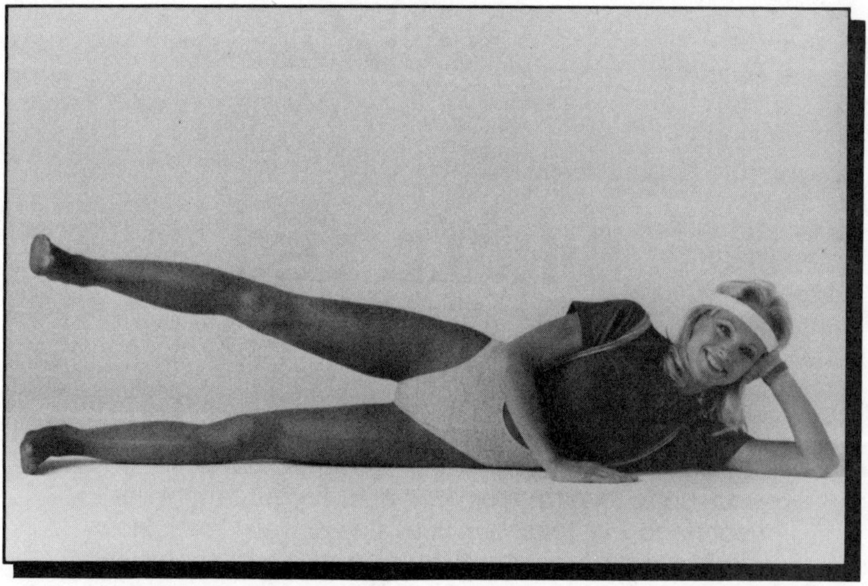

6

SINGLE LEG CROSSOVER

Lie on your back with your arms held out at your shoulders. Slowly raise your right leg up (toes pointed), pause and then lower it across your body toward your left hand. If you cannot reach your hand, just touch the floor at your waist level. Slowly return your leg to a straight-up position, and then slowly down to the starting position. Repeat with your left leg, right, left, etc. *Note:* Try to keep your head and upper body in contact with the floor as much as possible during the exercise.

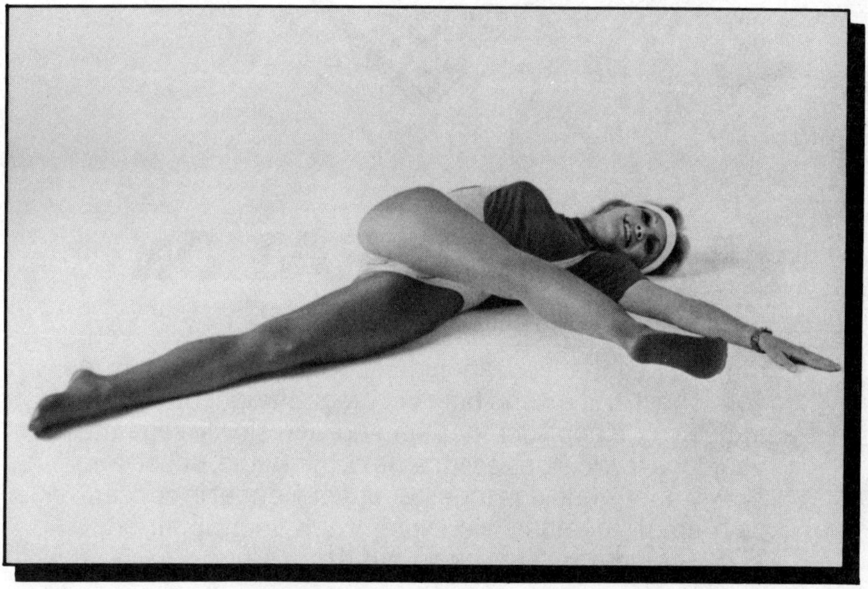

7

LEG SEPARATION

Lie on your back with your arms held out at your shoulders. Bend your knees up to your chest and extend both your legs straight up toward the ceiling. Keep your toes pointed, and slowly separate your legs to the sides as far as is comfortable, pause and slowly draw your legs together again. Repeat in succession apart, together, etc. *Note:* Keep your upper body and hips on the floor during the exercise.

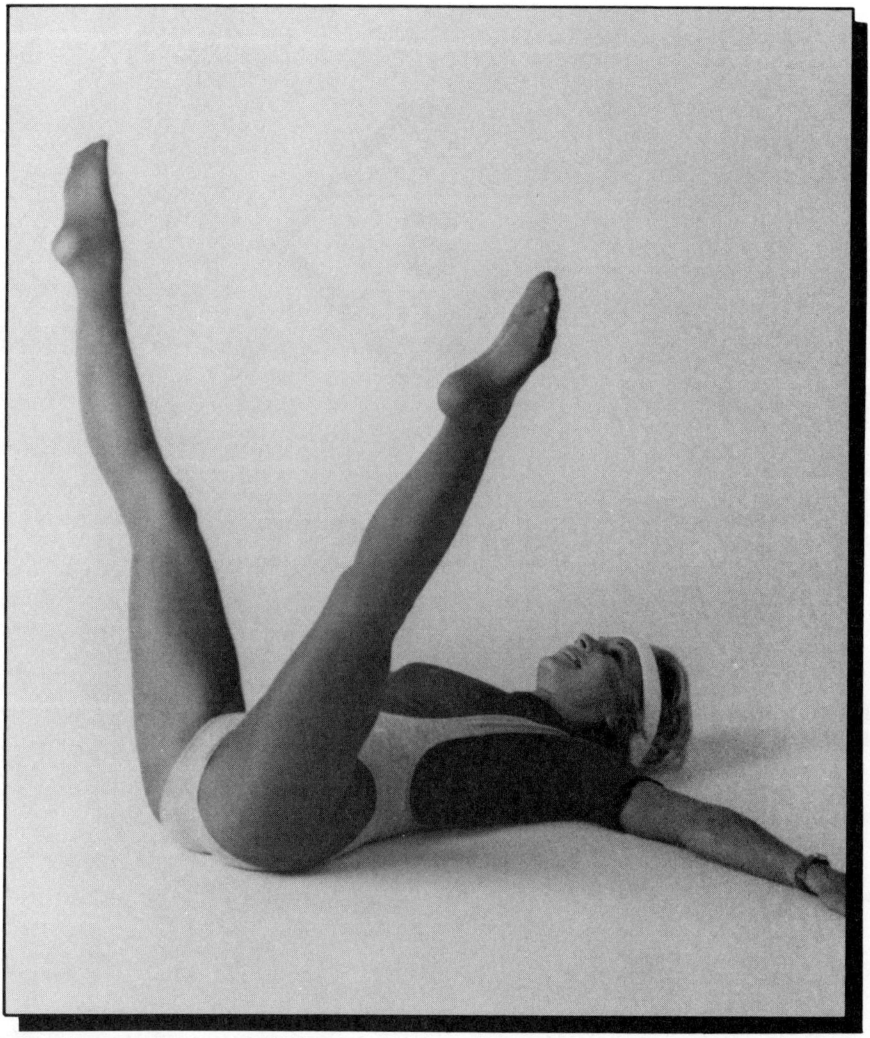

8

WALL SIT

Sit against a wall with your feet flat on the floor. Press your back, shoulders and head tight against the wall, resting your hands on your thighs. Hold this sitting position for 15 to 30 seconds and increase to one minute if possible. *Note:* Do not be surprised (especially if you are unaccustomed to exercise) if your thighs fatigue and even "tingle" after only 10 to 15 seconds of this exercise.

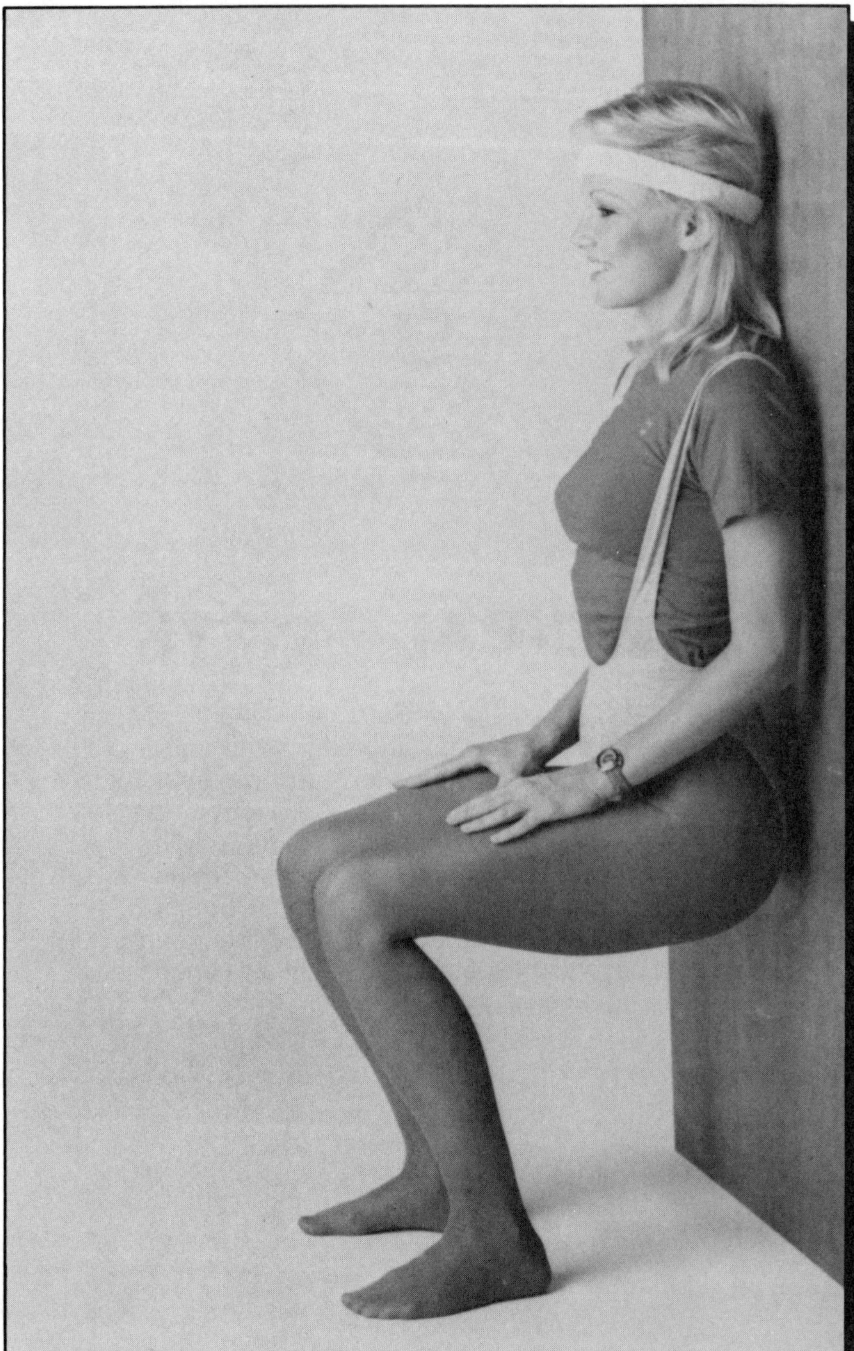

9

PLIÉ-CALF LIFTS

Stand with your legs apart, your feet pointed outward and your hands resting on your hips. Slowly bend your knees and lower your body slightly, then straighten your knees and quickly raise up onto your toes. Hold and then return to the starting position. Repeat lowering and lifting in succession. *Note:* Keep your head up and back straight. Also do not bend your knees too much—they should be directly over your toes, not beyond the toes, which could put unnecessary strain on the knees.

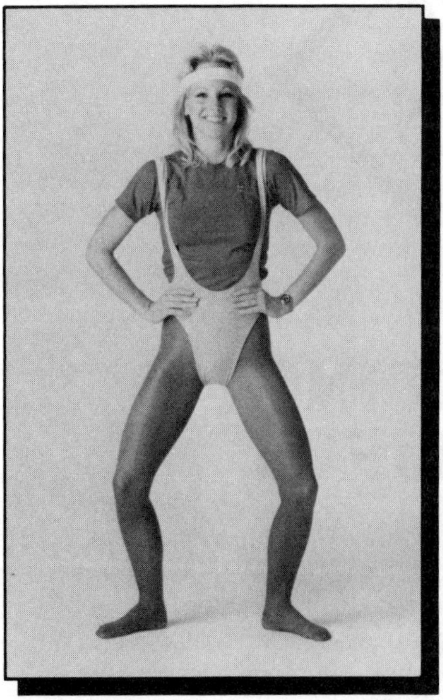

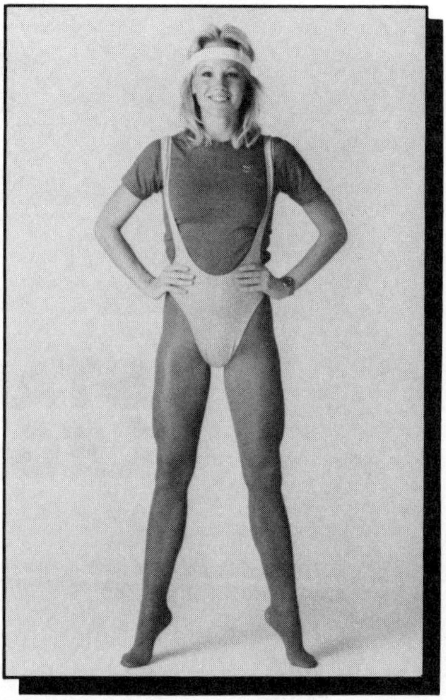

10

STANDING LEG LIFTS

Stand with your legs slightly apart and your left side to a wall or chair. With one hand on the wall or chair for balance, slowly lift your right leg forward (toes pointed), return to the starting position and continue the lift to the back (leaning slightly forward at the trunk). Return to the starting position and repeat lifting in succession forward, center, backward, center, etc. Repeat the exercise with the left leg. *Note:* keep your head up and your back as straight as possible while exercising.

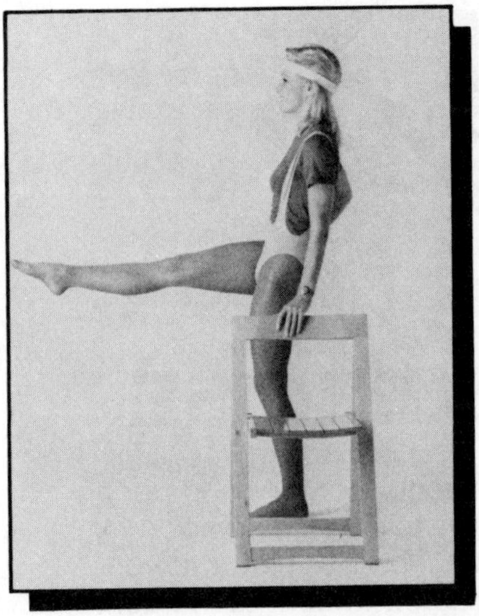

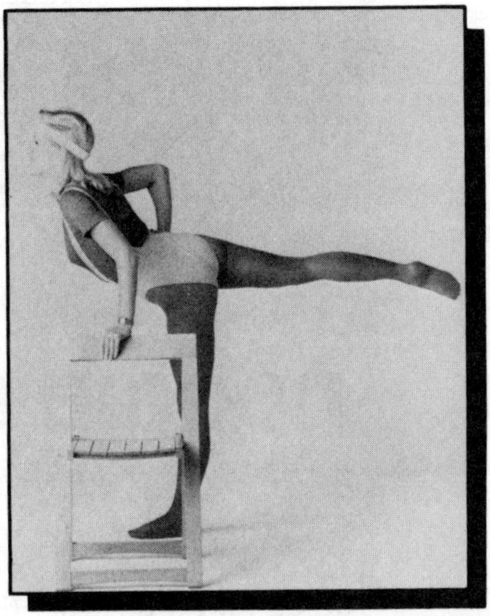

11

DOGGIE EXERCISE

Kneel on your hands and knees. Lift your left bent knee up to the side (Position 1), quickly extend your whole left leg straight out to your side as far as possible (Position 2), return to the bent knee position (Position 3), and back to the starting position (Position 4). Repeat with your right leg, left, right, etc. in succession. *Note:* Keep your head up during the exercise. Also keep your foot pointed up toward your shin while exercising.

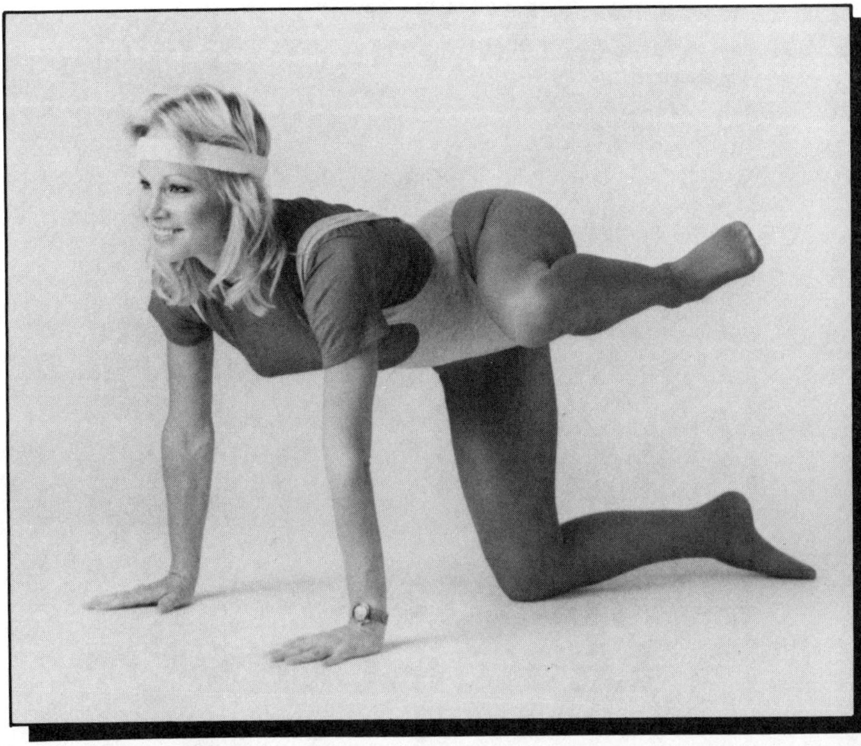

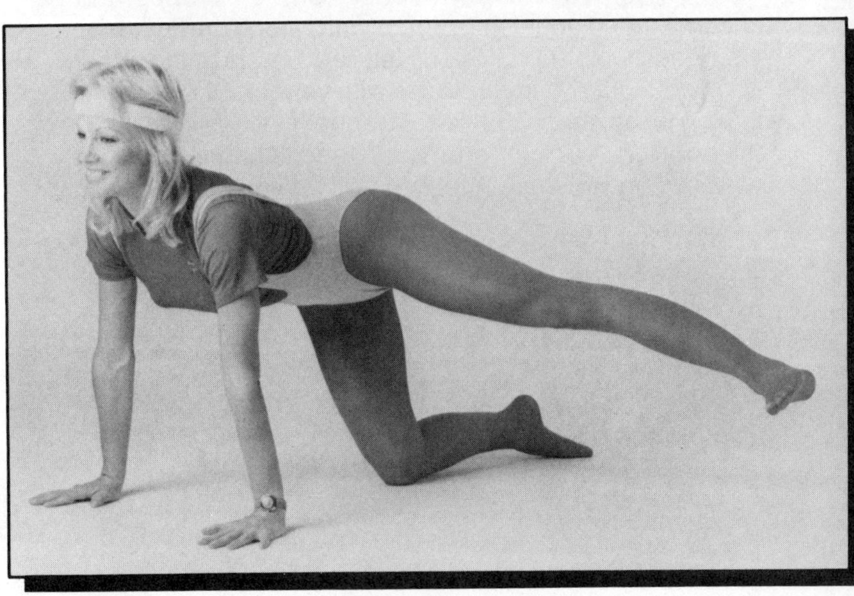

LEVEL II: INTERMEDIATE

12

HAND-KNEE LEG CIRCLES

Kneel on your hands and knees. Extend your left leg backward along the floor with your toes pointed. Lift your left leg up and hold. Now slowly describe 4 small circles with your foot. Lower your left leg to the starting position. Repeat the leg circles with the right leg, left, right, etc. *Note:* Keep your back straight while doing the leg circles, do not let your back sag if your legs tire.

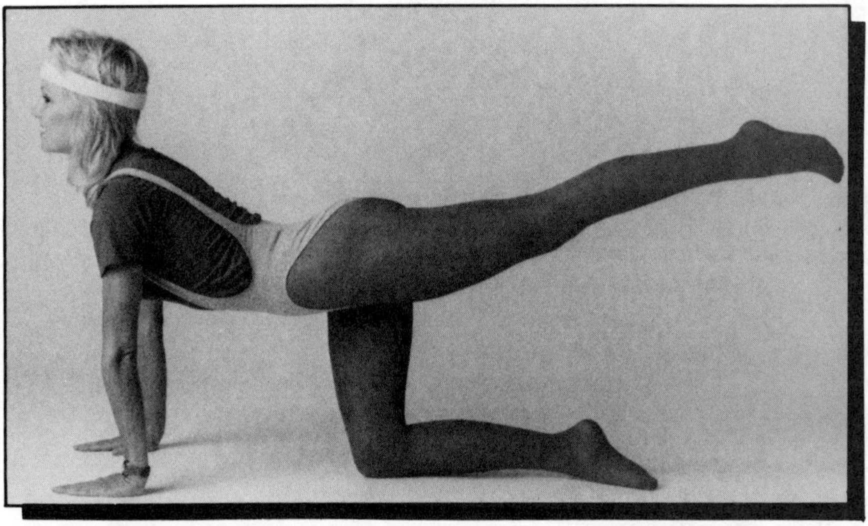

13

FLUTTER KICK

Lie on your stomach and place your head on your crossed arms in front of you. Point your toes, lift both legs up off the floor and flutter kick for 4 counts. Return your legs to the starting position, relax and repeat the kick. *Note:* Keep your head on your arms, do not bend your knees while kicking, and try not to arch your back. If this exercise bothers your back, do not do it!

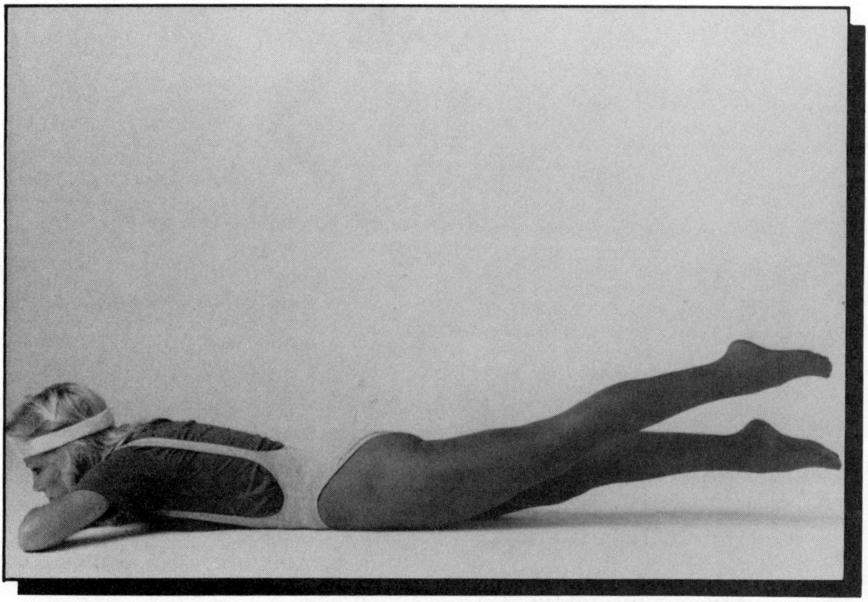

14

BICYCLE SEQUENCE

Sit back on the floor, supporting yourself up on your elbows. Lift both your legs up off the floor (only 12 to 15″) and slowly move your legs in a bicycle pedaling fashion for 4 counts. Relax and repeat pedaling. *Note:* Only bend your knees slightly while pedaling and do not arch your back.

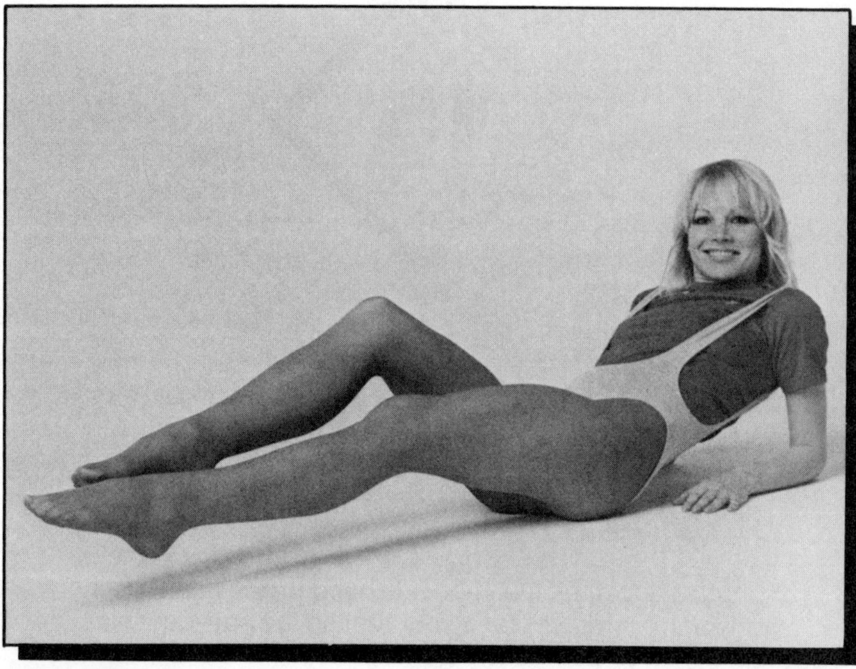

15

SIDE LYING DOUBLE LEG LIFT

Lie on your left side with one leg on top of the other, and one hand on the floor in front of you for support. Bend your feet up toward your shins. Slowly raise both legs up off the floor (10 to 12″), hold, and lower both legs to the starting position. Repeat lifting and lowering in succession. Repeat the exercise on your right side.

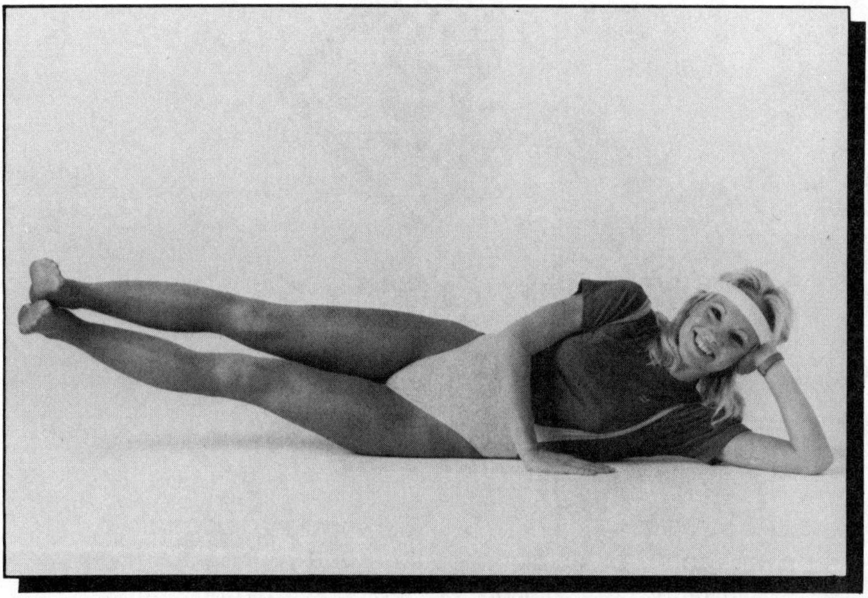

16

SIDE LYING INNER LEG LIFT

Lie on your left side with your left leg extended along the floor, and your right leg bent with your right foot on the floor behind your left knee. Place one hand on the floor in front of you for support. With your left foot bent up toward your shin, slowly lift your left leg up as far as possible, pause, and slowly lower it to the starting position. Repeat in succession. Repeat the exercise on the other side with the right leg. *Note:* Keep your body in a straight line on the floor while exercising—do not roll forward or backward.

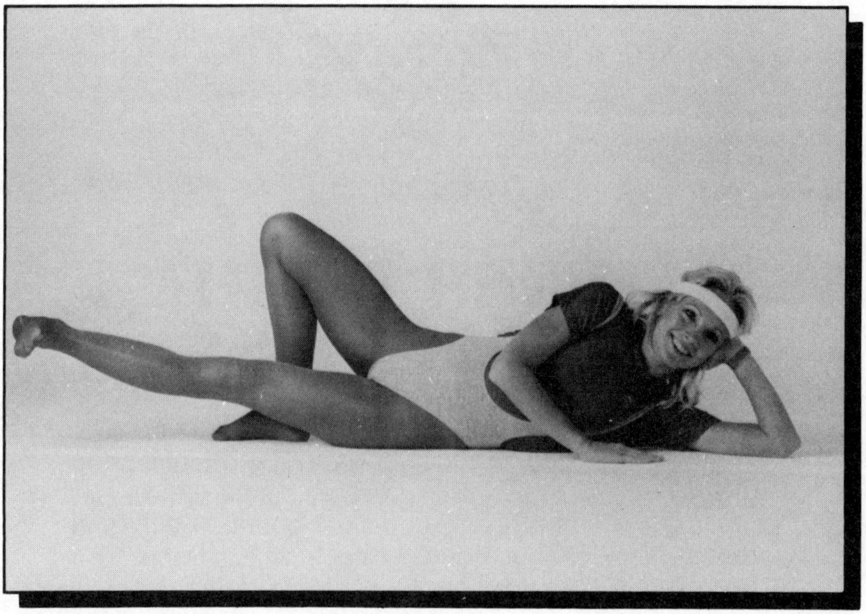

17

INNER THIGH CRISS-CROSS

Sit back on the floor, supporting yourself up on your elbows. Lift both your legs up off the floor (10 to 12″) with your toes pointed, and criss-cross your legs at the thighs for 4 counts. Relax and repeat. *Note:* Do not arch your back while exercising. If this exercise bothers your back, do not do it!

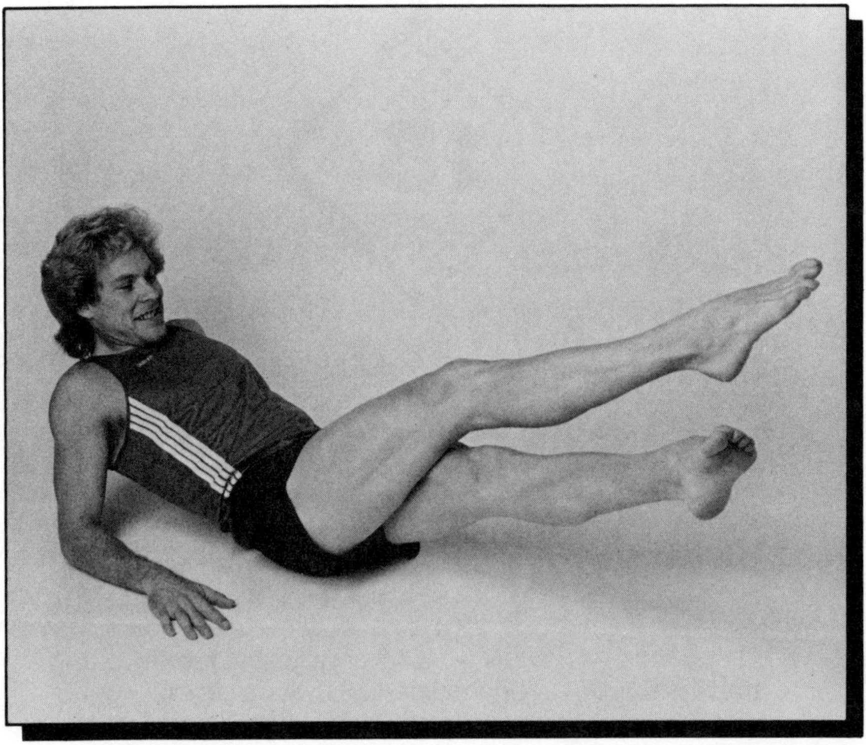

18

SINGLE LEG CROSSOVER VARIATION

Lie on your back with your arms held out at your shoulders. Slowly raise your right leg up (with your toes pointed), and lower it across your body toward your left hand. Hold your leg 1 to 2″ off the floor and slowly point your right foot forward and backward for 2 counts. Slowly return your leg to the straight up position and to the starting position. Repeat with your left leg, right, left, etc.

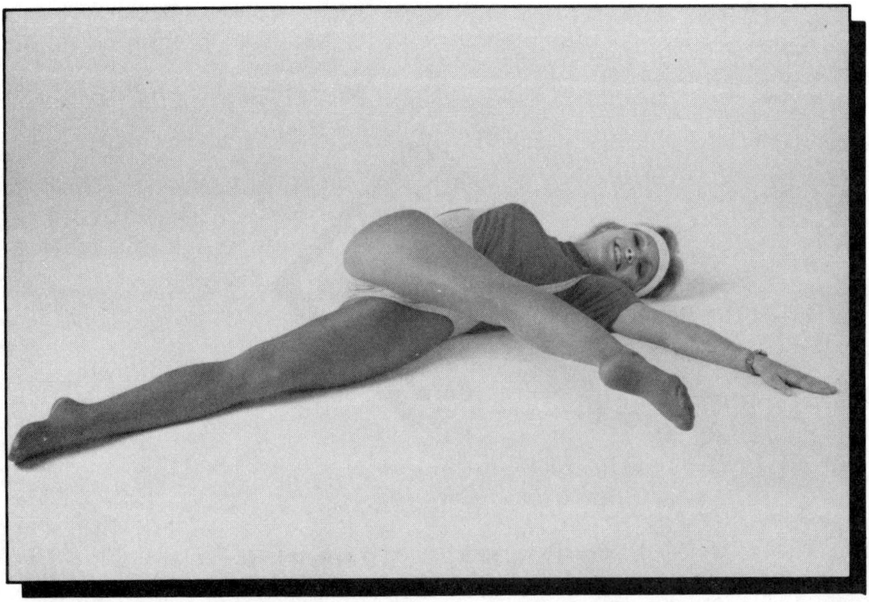

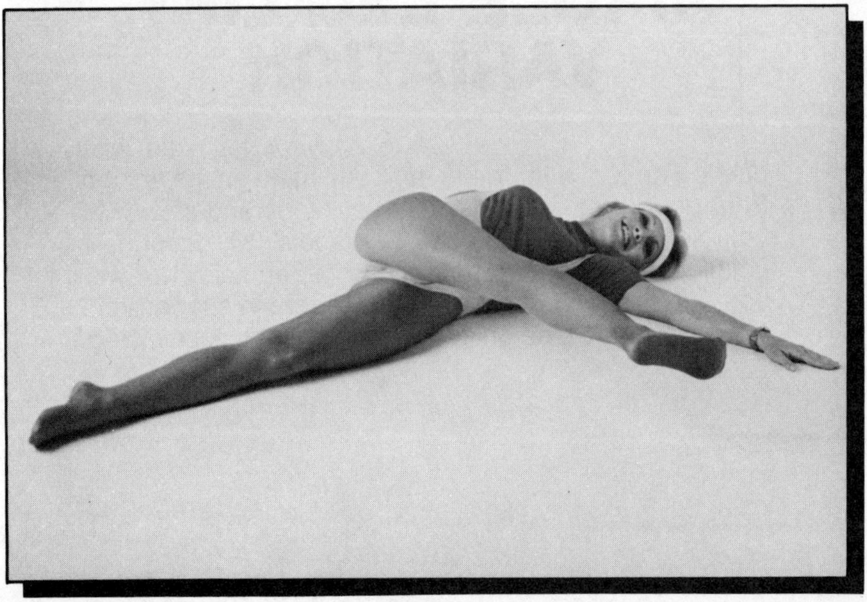

19

SIDE LYING SINGLE LEG LIFT VARIATION

Lie on your left side with one leg on top of the other, and one hand on the floor in front of you for support. Point your toes and slowly lift your right leg upward 8 to 10", hold and slowly describe 4 small circles with your right foot. Hold and slowly lower your leg to the starting position. Repeat in succession. Repeat the exercise on your other side with your left leg.

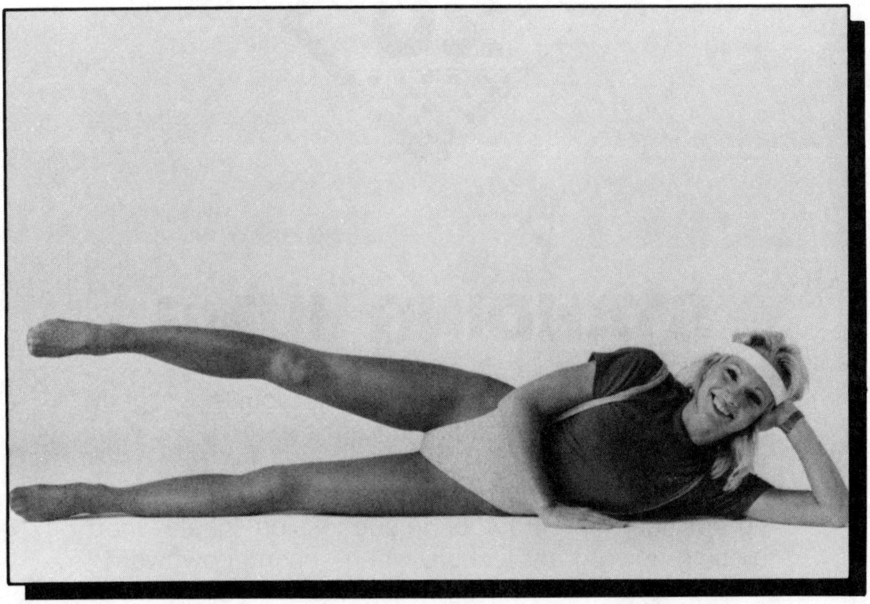

20

STANDING JUMP

Stand with your legs slightly apart, your knees bent and your arms extended at your sides. Jump vertically as high as possible (reaching upward with your arms) and return to the bent knee starting position. Repeat jumps in succession. Inhale when jumping upward and exhale when coming downward.

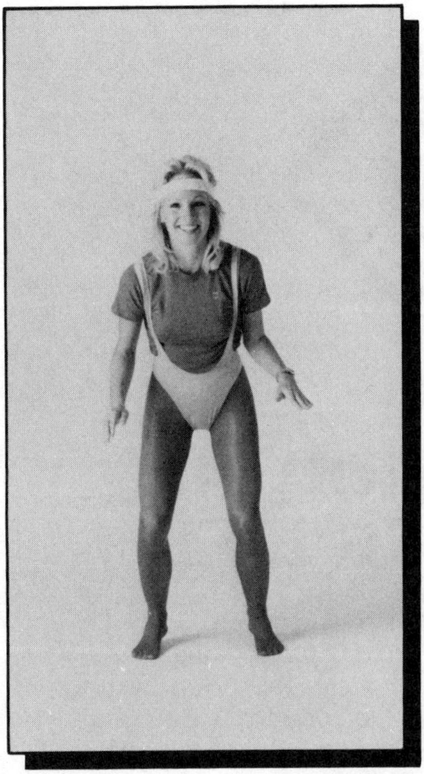

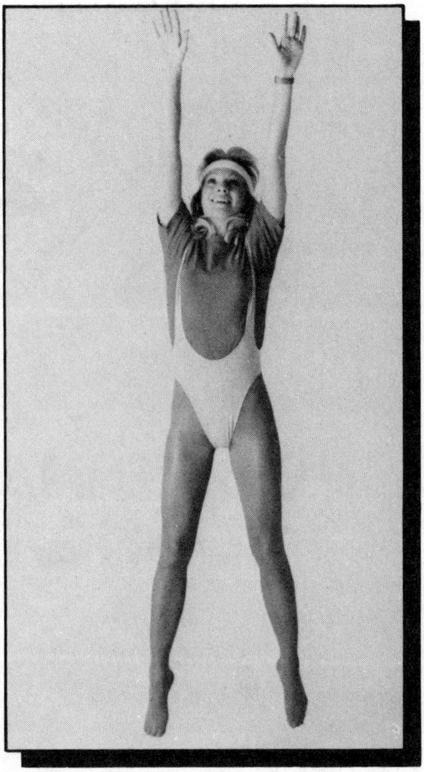

LEVEL III: ADVANCED

21

COMBINATION SIDE LYING LEG LIFT

Lie on your left side with one leg on top of the other, and one hand on the floor in front of you for support. With your toes pointed up toward your shins, slowly lift your right leg upward 8 to 10″ and hold. Now slowly lift your left leg up to touch your right leg, hold, and slowly lower both legs to the starting position. Repeat lifting and lowering your legs in succession. Repeat the exercise on your right side. *Note:* Be sure to keep your body in a straight line while exercising.

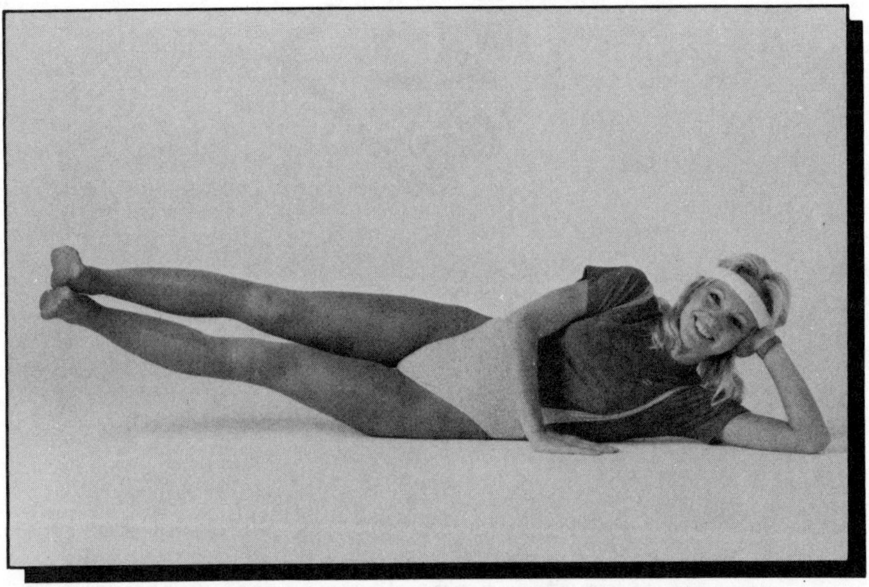

22

INNER THIGH CIRCLES

Sit back on the floor, supporting yourself up on your elbows. With your legs slightly apart, lift your right leg upward and with the heel of your foot (your toes are pointed up toward your shins) slowly describe 4 large circles. Return to the starting position, and repeat the exercise with the left leg, right, left, etc. *Note:* Describe as large a circle as possible 4 times without touching or resting the foot to the floor.

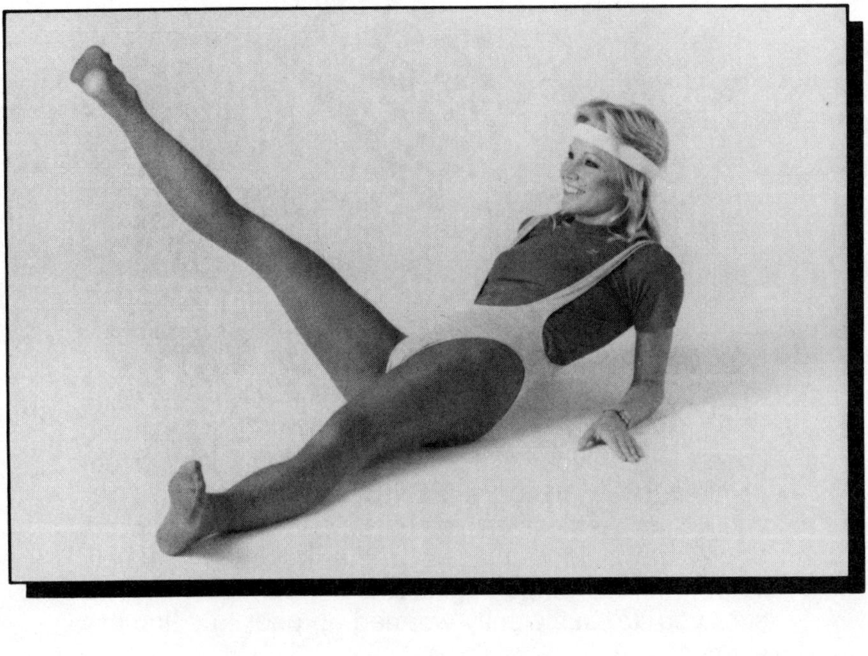

23

LATERAL LEG LIFT

Kneel on your hands and knees. Extend your left leg fully to the side with your foot pointed up toward your shin. Now slowly raise and lower your leg in succession. Repeat with the right leg. *Note:* Your leg should be placed on the floor approximately even with your supporting knee . . . not behind it. Also be sure you are sufficiently warmed up prior to doing this exercise!

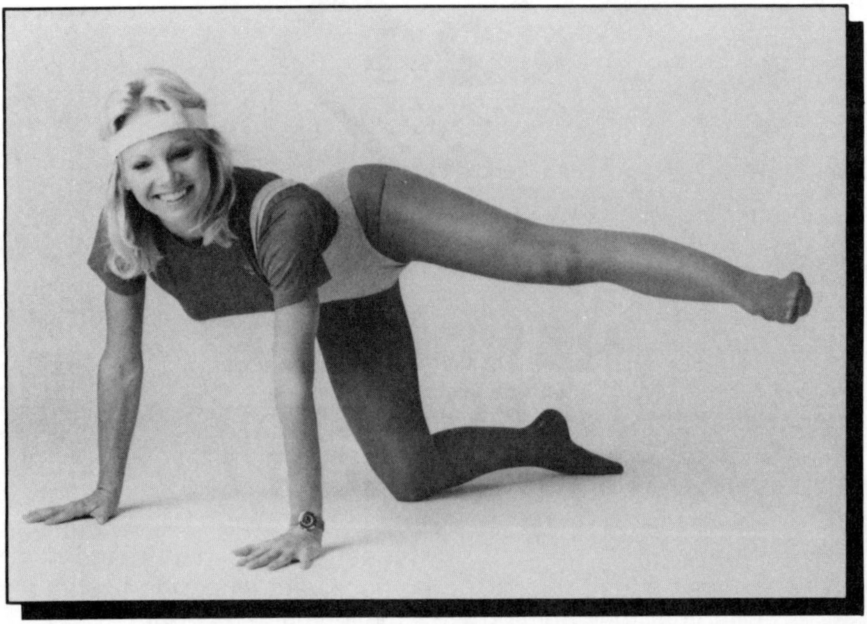

24

HAND-KNEE LEG LIFT VARIATION I

Kneel on your hands and knees. Extend your right leg backward along the floor with your toes pointed. Now move your leg about 10 to 12″ to your right and from that position, slowly lift and lower your leg in succession. Do *not* touch the floor or rest while doing the exercise. Repeat with the left leg placed 10 to 12″ to your left and again up off the floor. *Note:* Keep your head up and your back straight while exercising.

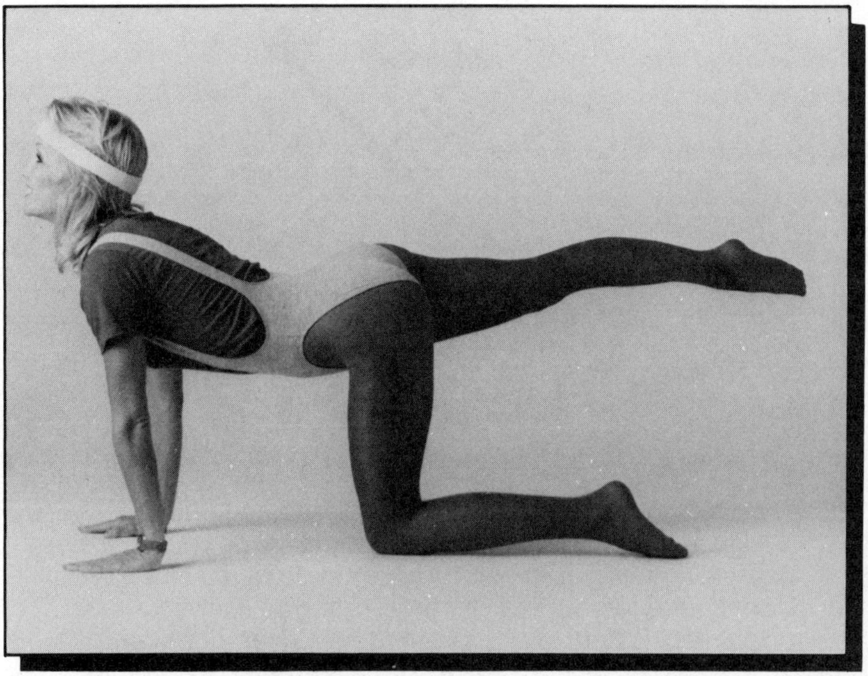

25

WALL SIT LEG LIFT

Sit against a wall with your feet flat on the floor. Press your head and upper body tight against the wall, and rest your hands on your thighs. Holding this position, lift your left knee up a few inches and extend your leg out in front of you with your toes pointed. Return your leg to the bent knee position and then lower your leg to the starting position. Repeat the leg lift with the right leg, left, right, etc. in succession. *Note:* Keep your back flat against the wall while doing the exercise.

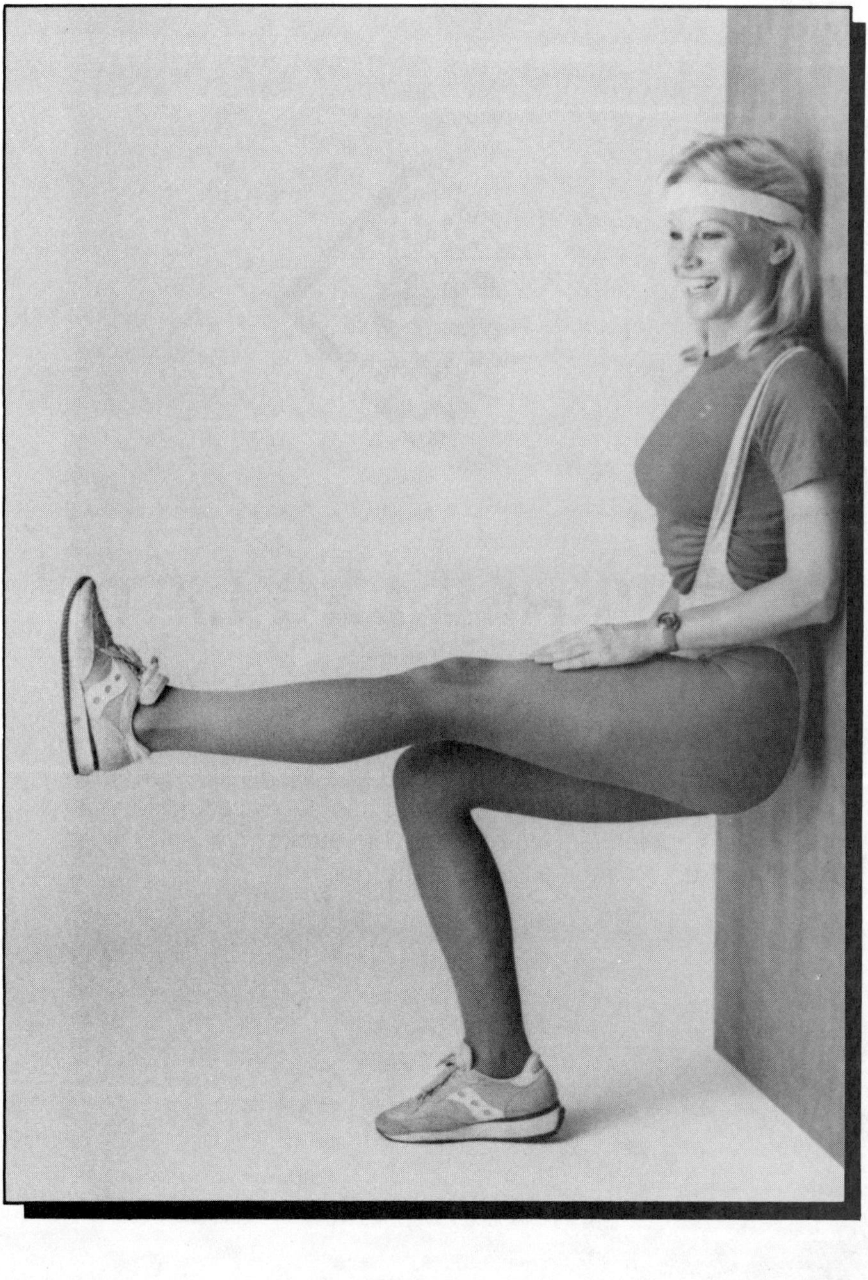

26

REVERSE LEG LIFT

Sit on the floor with your arms behind you. Now lift yourself up, supporting your weight on your hands and heels. Extend your right leg forward with your toes pointed and slowly lift your right leg above hip level, then lower it in succession. Repeat with your left leg. *Note:* Keep your back straight and hips held up so your back does not sag.

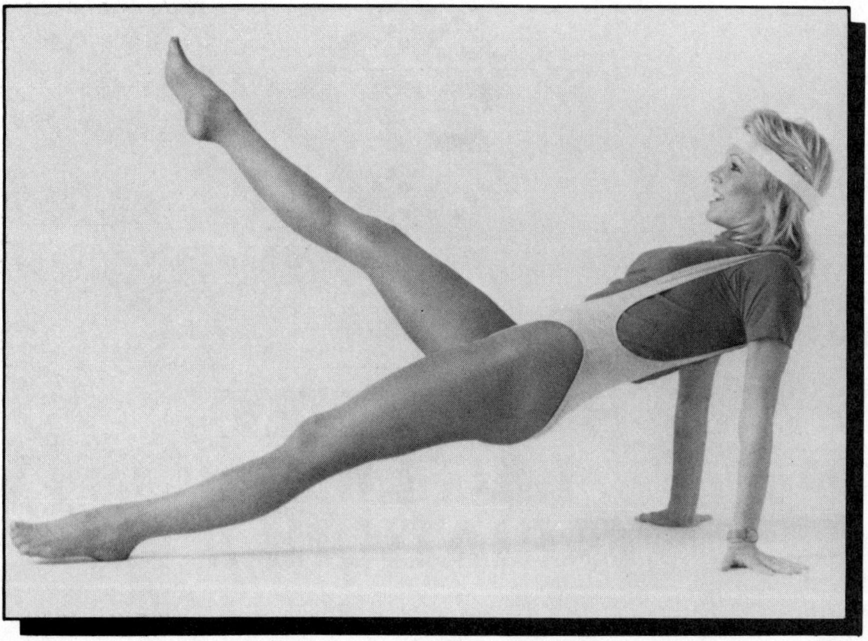

27

HAND-KNEE LEG LIFT VARIATION: II

Kneel on your hands and knees. Extend your left leg backward along the floor with your toes pointed. Now lift your left leg up and vigorously swing it to your left and back toward your right (behind your supporting right knee). Repeat in succession. Repeat the exercise with the right leg. *Note:* Keep your leg off the floor while swinging it right and left or left and right. Also keep your back straight and your head up.

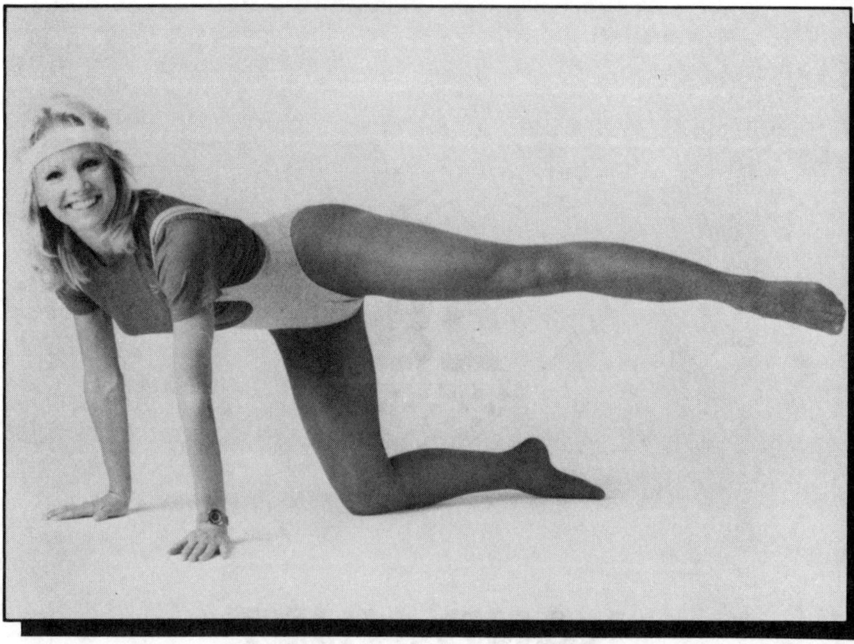

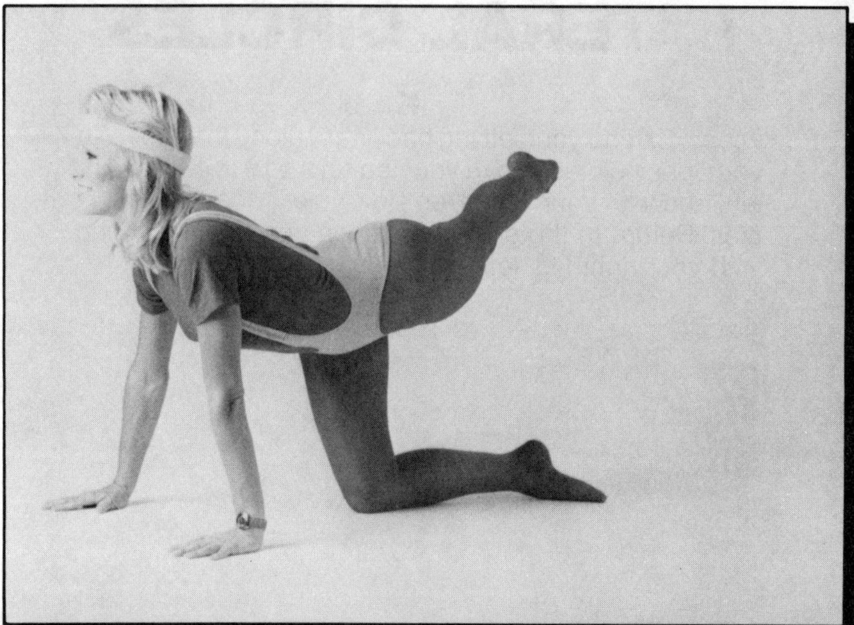

28

HAND-KNEE LATERAL CIRCLES

Kneel on your hands and knees. Extend your left leg backward along the floor with your toes pointed. Move your leg about 10 to 12″ to your left, and with your whole leg slowly describe 4 large circles. Return to the starting position and repeat circling with your right leg, left, right etc.

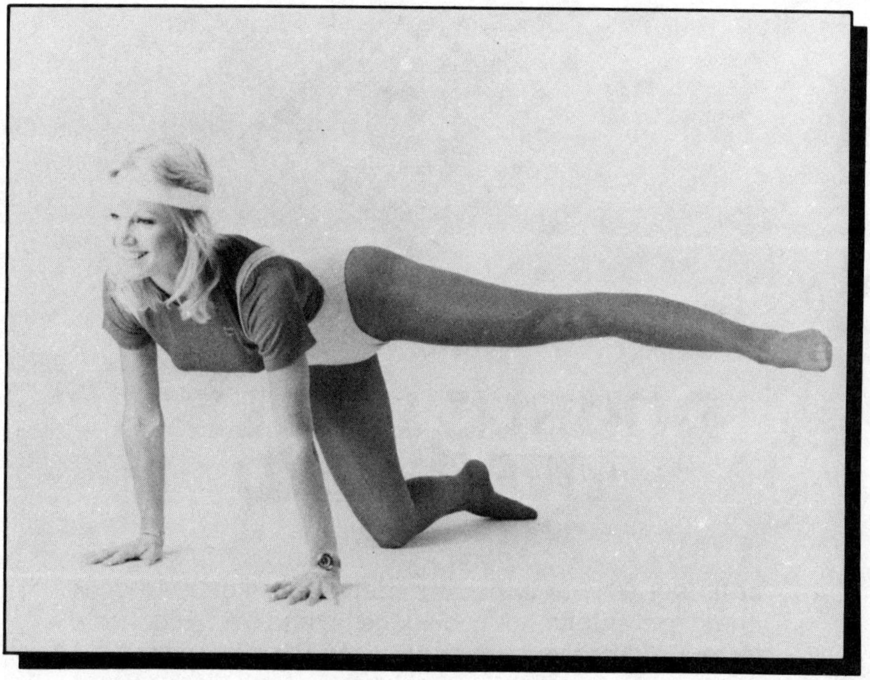

29

DOUBLE LEG LIFT OVERHEAD

Lie on your back with your arms out at your shoulders. Bend your knees to your chest and extend both your legs up and over your head to touch the floor with your toes. Then, placing your hands on your lower back, slowly lift both your legs up toward the ceiling with your toes pointed, and hold. Return to the knee-chest position, and to the floor or starting position. Relax and repeat. *Note:* Be sure that you are sufficiently warmed up prior to performing this exercise.

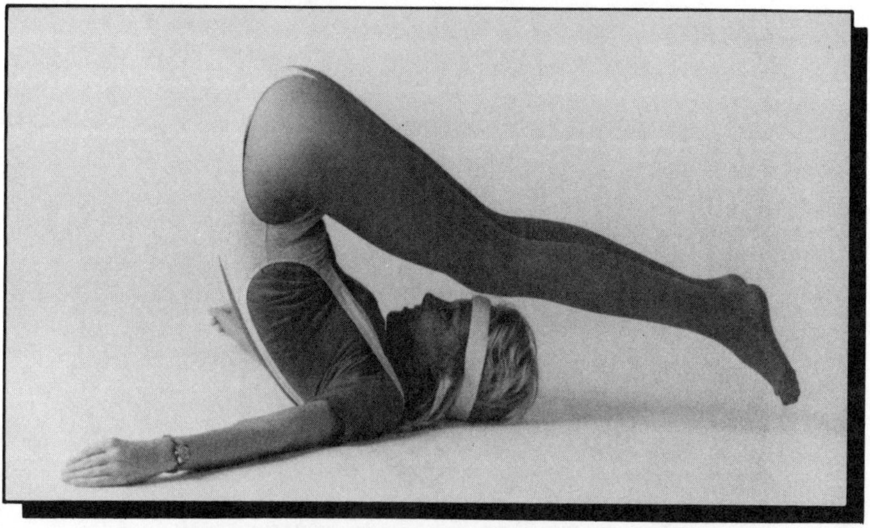

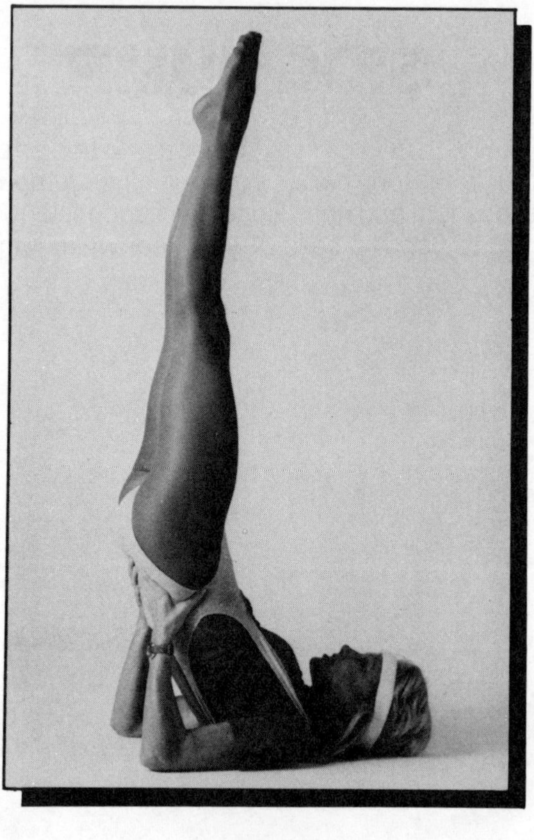

30

SIDE JUMP

Stand with your feet together and your hands on your hips. Jump forward, backward, left, and right. Repeat in succession. *Note:* Be sure to stay on the balls of your feet while jumping.

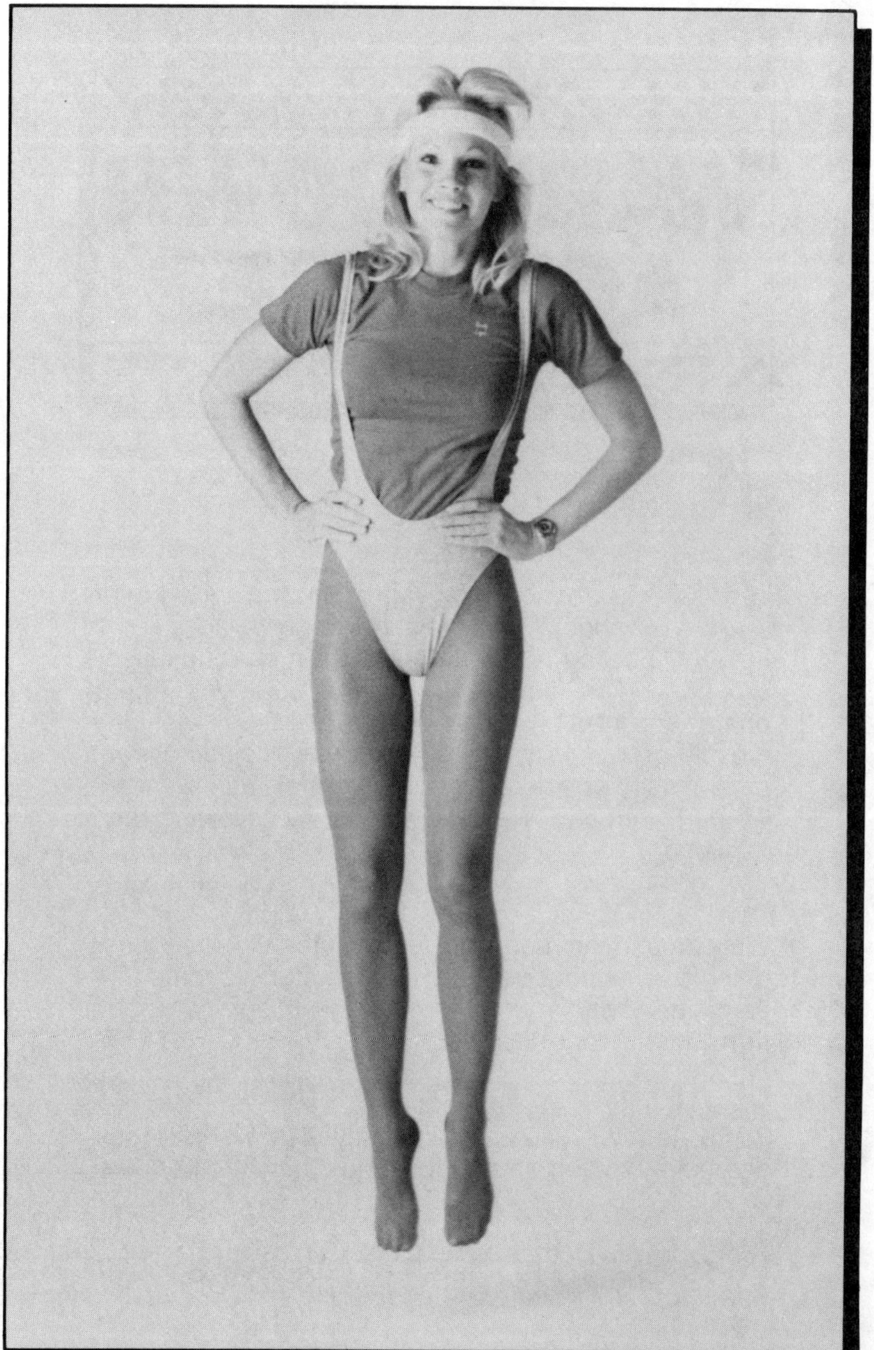

WARM-DOWN ACTIVITIES

After performing leg exercises, you should do a few warm-down activities to prevent "pooling" of waste products in specific muscle groups—which may cause muscle soreness. Appropriate activities should involve most of the large muscle groups in your body and may include a warm bath or shower. There are many possible activities from which to choose. We recommend the following (as a minimum):

1

Walk around the room for a few minutes, simultaneously doing a continuous series of exaggerated movements—step high, swing your arms, shake your legs, circle your arms, circle your head, etc.

2

Jump around, loosely shaking out your arms and legs—alternate jumping on one foot, the other, and both feet.

3

Repeat warm-up exercises #1 (Seated—Legs Together); #2 (Seated—Legs Apart)

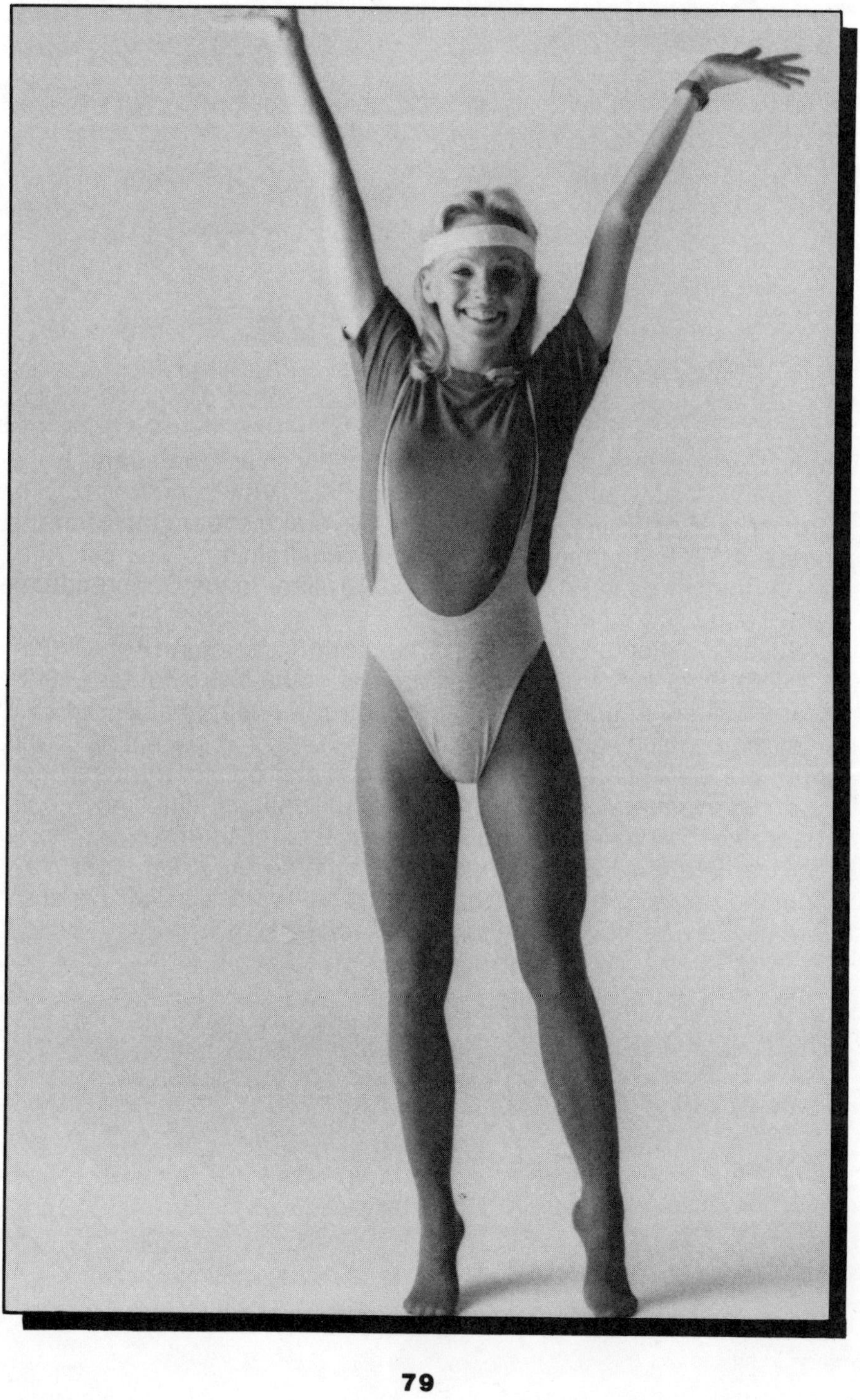

THE AUTHORS

Dr. James A. Peterson is the Director of Sports Medicine for the Women's Sports Foundation. The author of more than 20 books on sports and fitness, Dr. Peterson taught for over nine years at the United States Military Academy in West Point, New York. While on the faculty at West Point, he conducted several pioneer studies in the areas of strength training and the physical training of women. After West Point, he served as a fitness consultant to the Department of Athletics at Stanford University.

Susan L. Peterson is a free-lance writer who resides in Kensington, California. As the first woman instructor in the history of the United States Military Academy, she has appeared several times on national television, including the Johnny Carson Tonight Show. A fitness and self-defense expert, she has written several books and has been featured in several articles in national publications, including *People* magazine. The books she has authored include: *An Improved Figure Through Exercise, Self Defense for Women—The West Point Way, The Women's Stretching Book,* and *The Women's Self Defense Book—How to Stay Safe and Fight Back.*